# Guide to Learning Disabilities *for Primary Care*

## How to Screen, Identify, Manage, and Advocate for Children With Learning Disabilities

Larry B. Silver, MD
Life Fellow, AACAP
Clinical Professor of Psychiatry
Georgetown University Medical Center
Washington, DC

Dana L. Silver, MD, FAAP
The Herman and Walter Samuelson
Children's Hospital at Sinai
Baltimore, MD

American Academy of Pediarics
141 Northwest Point Blvd
Elk Grove Village, IL 60007-1098

**AAP Department of Marketing and Publications**

Maureen DeRosa, MPA, Director, Department of Marketing and Publications

Mark Grimes, Director, Division of Product Development

Diane Lundquist, Senior Product Development Editor

Sandi King, MS, Director, Division of Publishing and Production Services

Kate Larson, Manager, Editorial Services

Theresa Wiener, Manager, Publications Production and Manufacturing

Peg Mulcahy, Manager, Graphic Design and Production

Kevin Tuley, Director, Division of Marketing and Sales

Linda Smessaert, Manager, Clinical and Professional Publications Marketing

Library of Congress Control Number: 2010905153
ISBN: 978-1-58110-486-8
MA0561

9-273/0910

2  3  4  5  6  7  8  9  10

# Table of Contents

# Introduction

School is the "workplace" for children and adolescents. Successful school performance is essential for psychological and social growth. Lack of success might lead to emotional difficulties, peer problems, or social difficulties. It is for these reasons that pediatricians must inquire about school and school performance at every well-child visit and at acute care visits.

Difficulties in school can lead to stresses within the family. The earlier any weaknesses or disabilities are recognized and appropriate interventions begun, the better the outcome for the child. Without early identification and intervention, the academic problems compound each year, resulting in greater problems and in the child falling further behind. Equally important, these early interventions minimize the possibility of secondary emotional, social, and family problems.

In the office, a parent might discuss concerns with the child's behaviors in school and possibly at home. No mention might be made of academic difficulties. However, when the pediatrician asks, this parent might comment that their child is underachieving or poorly achieving in school. Not infrequently, the child first becomes an issue in school when the frustrations and lack of success lead to emotional or behavioral problems.

When the pediatrician is exploring why the child is underachieving or doing poorly in school, it is important to clarify if these emotional, social, and family problems are causing the academic difficulties or if the academic difficulties and the resulting feelings of frustration and failure are causing the emotional, social, and family problems. To treat the emotional problems resulting from unrecognized and untreated learning disabilities without identifying and addressing these disabilities will only result in lack of progress and in increased difficulties.

When a child is not successful in school, parents often turn to their general pediatrician for guidance. Yet many pediatricians do not have a clinical model for assessing why a patient might be struggling in school. The goal of this book is to provide pediatricians with the knowledge base and clinical skills to assess for and facilitate treatment for children who struggle in school. The assessment models to be discussed will fit within the time and personnel limits of a general practice of pediatrics.

Full or partial psychological or educational evaluations are neither necessary nor appropriate in a busy general pediatrician's office. Screening and referral for further evaluation is the goal, just as it is done with the early identification and referral for autism and other developmental disorders.

This book will focus on the most frequent cause of academic difficulties: learning disabilities. Many children with learning disabilities also have a language disability or a motor coordination disorder. Thus each of these disorders will be discussed as well as the office-based assessment process for each.

In recent years, the American Academy of Pediatrics has focused on the early recognition and diagnosis of developmental delay in children in the hope that early intervention will maximize the child's potential. This focus is also essential for children with the disabilities covered in this book. Early interventions maximize the child's ability to succeed academically by learning compensatory strategies and by receiving the necessary accommodations. Early intervention also decreases the child's experiences with frustration and failure.

The pediatrician, as child and family advocate, must play an essential role in assessing for and then helping the family find appropriate treatments for the child's learning, language, and/or motor disabilities. This supportive role starts with finding clinical evidence suggesting such disabilities. Next the pediatrician must play a supportive role during the evaluation process (interpreting the results of testing) and school intervention plans. It is important to help the family understand their child's strengths and weaknesses. Much as the school must build on the child's abilities while addressing the disabilities, the family must learn how to maximize the child's strengths and compensate for the child's weaknesses within the family, in social settings, and during activities. These plans must be adjusted for each phase of development. This book will cover each of these themes.

## Format of the Book

Part I focuses on each of these disabilities. Chapter 1 clarifies the differences between learning disorder and learning disabilities, Chapter 2 describes the types of learning disabilities a child might have, Chapter 3 focuses on the diagnosis of a learning disability, Chapter 4 focuses on language disabilities, Chapter 5 focuses on motor disabilities, and Chapter 6 focuses on the office-based assessment process to confirm each diagnosis and clarify the needs.

Part II addresses the disorders often associated with learning disabilities. Chapter 7 reviews the secondary emotional, social, and family problems. Chapter 8 introduces other primary disabilities often found with children who have learning disabilities. These comorbid conditions must be screened for as well. Chapter 9 addresses the social skills difficulties children with learning disabilities might have. This chapter will describe those social skills problems that are secondary to the learning, language, and/or motor deficits as well as the neurologically based pragmatic social skills problems often found with children who have learning disabilities.

Part III addresses the public school system. Chapter 10 focuses on important education laws, policies, and models of intervention as they relate to students with learning disabilities. The role of the pediatrician in facilitating essential assessments and interventions is emphasized. Chapter 11 goes into detail about the school assessment process and on the models of intervention for students with learning disabilities.

Part IV stresses the need for follow-up care. Most learning, language, and motor disabilities are life disabilities. They do not go away. Interventions, thus, will change with age and grade. Chapter 12 focuses on interventions for the primary comorbid disorders and Chapter 13 addresses the secondary emotional, social, and family problems.

Part V consists of Appendix A, a listing relevant organizations and other resources for health professionals and for patients and their families; Appendix B, a compilation of reproducible screening forms.

The general pediatrician is the primary advocate for the child and the family. Our goal and only purpose for writing this book is to expand the pediatrician's ability to be the primary advocate for the child and family when the presenting problems relate to academic or behavioral difficulties in school. We wish to empower the pediatrician with the skills to do this in a relatively quick and efficient office-based manner.

# PART I

# Learning and Related Disabilities

# Chapter 1

#  *Learning Disorders Versus Learning Disabilities*

Learning disabilities are neurologically based disorders resulting from incorrect or faulty wiring of neurons in the brain. Language disabilities and motor disabilities are also neurologically based and also result from incorrect or faulty wiring of neurons in the brain. Thus, based on where the neurologically based problems occur in the brain, a child will have a learning, language, and/or motor disorder.

The medical terms used for learning difficulties are based on the *International Classification of Diseases (ICD)*. In the United States, this section of the *ICD* is found in the *Diagnostic and Statistical Manual of Mental Disorders (DSM)*. Here, the term *learning disorders* is used. When completing forms for insurance companies, these medical terms must be used.

The educational systems within the United States are guided by US federal law and the term *learning disabilities* is used. When writing reports for a public school system or when communicating with public school professionals, the term *learning disabilities* should be used.

In clinical practice it is important to understand the medical and the educational terms. The medical term *learning disorders* will be discussed first.

## Learning Disorders

The current edition of the *Diagnostic and Statistical Manual of Mental Disorders, Fourth Edition (DSM-IV)* was published in 1994. Based on field trials and new research data, the text in this edition was modified in 2000 as *DSM-IV-TM*. It is based on the *International Statistical Classification of Diseases and Related Health Problems, Tenth Edition (ICD-10)*.

The term used for neurologically based academic difficulties is *learning disorders*. Several subtypes are noted: reading disorders, mathematics disorder, disorder of written expression, and learning disorder not otherwise specified. Two other groups of relevant problems are classified within this section of *DSM-IV-TM*: motor skills disorder and communication disorders.

---

### Diagnostic Criteria for Reading Disorder

A. Reading achievement, as measured by individually administered standardized tests of reading accuracy or comprehension, is substantially below that expected given the person's chronological age, measured intelligence, and age-appropriate education.

B. The disturbance in Criterion A significantly interferes with academic achievement or activities of daily living that require reading skills.

C. If a sensory deficit is present, the reading difficulties are in excess of those usually associated with it.

---

### Diagnostic Criteria for Mathematics Disorder

A. Mathematical ability, as measured by individually administered standardized tests, is substantially below that expected given the person's chronological age, measured intelligence, and age-appropriate education.

B. The disturbance in Criterion A significantly interferes with academic achievement or activities of daily living that require mathematical ability.

C. If a sensory deficit is present, the difficulties in mathematical ability are in excess of those usually associated with it.

---

### Diagnostic Criteria for Disorder of Written Expression

A. Writing skills, as measured by individually administered standardized tests (or functional assessments of writing skills), are substantially below those expected given the person's chronological age, measured intelligence, and age-appropriate education.

B. The disturbance in criterion A substantially interferes with academic achievement or activities of daily living that require the composition of written texts (eg, writing grammatically correct sentences and organized paragraphs).

C. If a sensory deficit is present, the difficulties in writing skills are in excess of those usually associated with it.

---

Each of these disorders is defined as difficulties in a specific academic area that are substantially below that expected, given the person's chronological age, measured intelligence, and age-appropriate education.

## Learning Disorders Not Otherwise Specified

This category is for disorders in learning that do not meet criteria for any specific learning disorders, for example, a disorder in which spelling skills are substantially below those expected given the person's chronological age, measured intelligence, and age-appropriate education. Because the *DSM-IV-TM* diagnostic categories do not recognize such higher learning skills as organization and executive function, disabilities in these areas are often coded under this heading.

## Disorders Often Found When the Child Has a Learning Disability

Children who have learning disabilities might also have difficulties with motor skills and/or with language skills. Each of these possible comorbid disorders will be noted as they are found in *DSM-IV*.

### Motor Skills Disorder

Only one category is listed, developmental coordination disorder.

---

**Diagnostic Criteria for Developmental Coordination Disorder**

A. Performance in daily activities that require motor coordination is substantially below that expected given the person's chronological age and measured intelligence. This may be manifested by marked delays in achieving motor milestones (eg, walking, crawling, sitting), dropping things, "clumsiness," poor performance in sports, or poor handwriting.

B. The disturbance in Criterion A significantly interferes with academic achievement or activities of daily living.

C. The disturbance is not due to a general medical condition (eg, cerebral palsy, hemiplegia, or muscular dystrophy) and does not meet criteria for a pervasive developmental disorder.

D. If mental retardation is present, the motor difficulties are in excess of those usually associated with it.

---

Reprinted from: American Psychiatric Association: *Diagnostic and Statistical Manual of Mental Disorders*, Fourth Edition, Text Revision. Washington DC: American Psychiatric Association; 2000:58.

## *Communication Disorders*

Subgroups reflect either difficulties processing oral language or speech production. This book will focus on the language-based communication disorders only.

---

### Diagnostic Criteria for Expressive Language Disorder

A. The scores obtained from standardized individually administered measures of expressive language development are substantially below those obtained from standardized measures of both nonverbal intellectual capacity and receptive language development. The disturbance may be manifested clinically by symptoms that include having a markedly limited vocabulary, making errors in tense, or having difficulty recalling words or producing sentences with developmentally appropriate length or complexity.

B. The difficulties with expressive language interfere with academic or occupational achievement or with social communication.

C. Criteria are not met for Mixed Receptive-Expressive Language Disorder or a Pervasive Developmental Disorder.

D. If Mental Retardation, a speech-motor or sensory deficit, or environmental deprivation is present, the language difficulties are in excess of those usually associated with these problems.

---

### Diagnostic Criteria for Mixed Receptive-Expressive Language Disorder

A. The scores obtained from a battery of standardized individually administered measures of both receptive and expressive language development are substantially below those obtained from standardized measures of nonverbal intellectual capacity. Symptoms include those for Expressive Language Disorder as well as difficulty understanding words, sentences, or specific types of words, such as spatial terms.

B. The difficulties with receptive and expressive language significantly interfere with academic or occupational achievement or with social communication.

C. Criteria are not met for a Pervasive Developmental Disorder.

D. If Mental Retardation, a speech-motor or sensory deficit, or environmental deprivation is present, the language difficulties are in excess of those usually associated with these problems.

---

Reprinted from: American Psychiatric Association: *Diagnostic and Statistical Manual of Mental Disorders*, Fourth Edition, Text Revision. Washington DC: American Psychiatric Association; 2000:61, 64.

Several diagnostic categories in *DSM-IV-TR* are not directly relevant to this book. They are listed to reflect the full categories of communication disorders.

---

### Diagnostic Criteria for Phonological Disorders

A.  Failure to use developmentally expected speech sounds that are appropriate for age and dialect (eg, errors in sound production, use, representation, or organization such as, but not limited to, substitutions of one sound for another [use of /t/ for target /k/ sound] or omissions of sounds such as final consonants).

B.  The difficulties in speech sound production interfere with academic or occupational achievement or with social communication.

C.  If Mental Retardation, a speech-motor or sensory deficit, or environmental deprivation is present, the speech difficulties are in excess of those usually associated with these problems.

---

### Stuttering

A.  Disturbance in the normal fluence and time patterning of speech (inappropriate for the individual's age) characterized by frequent occurrences of one or more of the following:
    (1) sound and syllable repetitions
    (2) sound prolongations
    (3) interjections
    (4) broken words (eg, pauses within a word)
    (5) audible or silent blocking (filled or unfilled pauses in speech)
    (6) circumlocution (word substitutions to avoid problematic words)
    (7) words produced with excess of physical tension
    (8) monosyllabic whole-word repetitions (eg, "I-I-I-I see him")

B.  The disturbance in fluency interferes with academic or occupational achievement or with social communication.

C.  If a speech-motor or sensory deficit is present, the speech difficulties are in excess of those usually associated with these problems.

---

Reprinted from: American Psychiatric Association: *Diagnostic and Statistical Manual of Mental Disorders,* Fourth Edition, Text Revision. Washington DC: American Psychiatric Association; 2000:66, 69.

## *Communication Disorder Not Otherwise Specified*

This category is for disorders in communication that do not meet criteria for any specific communication disorder; for example, a voice disorder (ie, an abnormality of vocal pitch, loudness, quality, tone, or resonance).

# *Learning Disabilities*

In 1975 the US Congress considered a groundbreaking education law. For the first time in the United States, the need for public education for all children, including those with disabilities, was addressed. Prior to this law, public school systems were not required to recognize or address the needs of children with disabilities. Since the intent of this law was to address the needs of children with disabilities, the organizations involved in working with children who had neurologically based learning problems decided that to ensure their children were included in this law, the name for these problems had to be *learning disabilities.*

The federal definition of learning disabilities is based on this initial law defining learning problems as a disability and clarifying what public schools must do to address these disabilities. The initial law was passed in 1975 by the US Congress and called The Education for all Handicapped Children Act. Since it was the 142nd law passed by the 94th Congress, the law is often referred to as Public Law 94-142. Over time, the name of this law was changed to Individuals with Disabilities Education Act (IDEA). Congress has revised this law over the years. The most recent revision, in 2004, changed the name of the law to the Individuals with Disabilities Education and Improvement Act; however, it is still referred to as IDEA 2004. Throughout these changes in the law, the definition of a learning disability remained as stated in 1975.

> *Specific learning disabilities* means a disorder in one or more of the basic psychological processes involved in understanding or in using language, spoken or written, which may manifest itself in an imperfect ability to listen, think, speak, read, write, spell, or to do mathematical calculations. The term includes such conditions as perceptual handicaps, brain injury, minimal brain dysfunction, dyslexia, and developmental aphasia. The term does not include children who have learning problems which are primarily the result of visual, hearing, or motor handicaps, or mental retardation, of emotional disturbance, or of environmental, cultural, or economic disadvantage.

This definition specifically states that the underlying deficits relate to processing problems. It also clarifies that these deficits are not caused by other neurologically based disorders (visual, hearing, or motor handicaps; mental retardation). Nor are these deficits the result of emotional, environmental, cultural, or economic difficulties.

## Medical Versus Educational Definitions

The medical definition, *learning disorder,* stresses a deficit in a specific academic skill. The educational definition, *learning disability,* stresses the neurologic basis for the disabilities and places the focus not just on the specific skill involved, but also on the underlying processing problems.

The purpose for a diagnosis is that it helps clarify the necessary interventions to address the diagnosis. It also is necessary in terms of *ICD-9-CM* and *Current Procedural Terminology* coding and payment for the physician. Using a diagnostic term that only identifies an area of skill deficit is not as useful as using a term that clarifies the neurologic basis for the deficit and that leads to an intervention plan. It is this knowledge of areas of neurologically based processing strengths and deficits that assist in developing the most effective treatment interventions.

Because processing disorders may affect more than one learning skill, it is not uncommon for a child to have learning disabilities in more than one area. It is important for the pediatrician to understand this concept and to explore all areas of learning when assessing the child.

## Bibliography

American Psychiatric Association. *Diagnostic and Statistical Manual of Mental Disorders.* 4th ed. Text rev. Washington, DC: American Psychiatric Association; 1994

Latham PS, Latham H, Mandlewitz M. *Special Education Law.* Washington, DC: JKL Communications; 2008

World Health Organization. *Classification of Diseases.* 10th rev. Clin mod. Geneva, Switzerland: World Health Organization; 2003

Wright PWD, Wright PD. *Special Education Law.* 2nd ed. Hartfield, VA: Harbor House Law Press; 2008

# Chapter 2

*Learning Disabilities*

---

Mrs Weaver visits your office in November with her 10-year-old son, Alex, who is in the fifth grade. She is concerned that he is misbehaving in school. He resists doing class work. When given an assignment by his teacher, he doodles or walks around the room. Alex also resists doing his homework. His teacher suggests that he might have an attentional disorder. You start by exploring the possible diagnosis of attention-deficit/hyperactivity disorder (ADHD).

---

Your discussions with Alex, his mother, and later with his teacher reveal that Alex can be active in class and that he can be inattentive. However, these behaviors only relate to doing desk work where he must read the instructions and perform the requested task in writing. During times when his teacher reads a story and asks for comments, he is very focused and often volunteers answers. You ask about home life. His mother describes the motor activity or inattention at home only when he is asked to do his schoolwork. His medical history is noncontributory. You ask for educational history and learn that his preschool, kindergarten, and first- and second-grade teachers never described Alex as overactive or inattentive. Although there is a family history on his mother's side of academic difficulties, there is no family history suggestive of ADHD. Since you establish neither a chronic nor a pervasive history of hyperactivity, inattention, or impulsivity, you feel comfortable ruling out ADHD. What next? Does he have behavioral problems? His mother reports no history of anxiety, depression, or anger control. She says that he is delightful at home and relates well to his friends. He has never been a behavioral problem in school. He appears not to have any apparent emotional or social difficulties. You next wonder if he might have a learning disability. How would you systematically explore for this diagnostic possibility?

The diagnostic process taught in medical school and used in the general pediatric residency is the medical model for assessing clinical problems. The presenting problem (chief complaint) triggers an organized model for data collection. A history of present illness is collected, which leads to a review of past, family, and/or social history. Questions based on an organized model for review of systems cover all relevant areas. The physical examination adds further clinical data. When needed, relevant clinical laboratory, imaging, or other studies lead to a diagnosis. This diagnosis then leads to a medical treatment plan.

Unique to the practice of pediatrics is the developmental model as it relates to each phase of the assessment. Not only are data collected, but these data are compared with where the child should be for his or her age. Are the findings age-appropriate, delayed, or above the expected level?

As noted in the introduction to this book, the American Academy of Pediatrics has recently emphasized the importance for early recognition and diagnosis of developmental delays in children. Early diagnosis and treatment is essential to maximize growth and success and to minimize frustrations and failures.

If the presenting problems are that the patient is not succeeding in school, some general pediatricians may do (or have someone else in the office do) an informal screening test to see if there might be a reading or writing problem. The next step would be to collect more information by asking questions using a review of systems model that focuses on education and learning. To do this, the pediatrician will need a developmental model for comparing the educational data collected with where the child should be for his age or grade. What are the developmental steps in learning to read, to write, or to do math? What should be mastered in preschool, first grade, third grade, fifth grade, middle school, or high school?

The data collected might suggest that the school problems are related to a problem with learning. With an educational developmental model, the pediatrician will know what questions to ask. Knowing normative data for age and grade, the pediatrician will be able to assess if the child is at grade level or below grade level for each expected academic skill. This information will lead to the necessary studies to clarify both in the office and elsewhere if the child has a learning disability. The final diagnosis will then lead to a medical treatment plan.

Before elaborating on an educational developmental model for doing a review of systems, it is important to review the aspects of an assessment already known to the pediatrician. These include knowledge of risk factors for learning problems and relevant family history that would increase the suspicion of a learning disability. The pediatrician's long-term contact with a child, frequently starting at birth, providing knowledge of the family and of family history plus developmental and medical history, is critical to suspecting the possibility of a learning, language, or motor disability.

## Risk Factors

### Medical History

These risk factors include a history of medical problems, family history, and the child's school history. A child with a history of premature delivery and/ or low birth weight should be considered at risk for academic difficulties and screened for such problems each year. If he or she has a history of head injury, a seizure disorder, lead poisoning, history of chemotherapy or radiation therapy for cancer, or a chronic health condition, the child is at greater risk of showing academic difficulties. Screening for possible school problems should be done each year.

Maternal alcohol or drug use during pregnancy, especially during the first trimester of pregnancy, is a high risk factor for brain-based disorders. A history of complications or medical problems during pregnancy as well as evidence of problems at delivery, especially those causing fetal distress, should be seen as risk factors.

Was the child adopted? If so, what were the circumstances? Most children who are adopted come from healthy parents who received good prenatal care. Was this true with the child being assessed? Children adopted from specific countries around the world often are at more risk for neurologically based problems. If the child is a product of a foreign adoption, is there a possibility that a parent was alcoholic or used drugs? Was there malnutrition? Abuse? Did the child spend time in an orphanage with minimal or poor attention or care? In addition to these concerns about the adoptive family and early child care, is there a history of either birth parent having academic or behavioral difficulties? Did the birth mother receive adequate prenatal care? Have adequate nutrition during pregnancy?

## Family and Social History

The traditional review of family history might identify possible risk factors. Does either parent have a history of academic difficulties? Did either have learning disabilities and/or ADHD as a child? How far did they go in school and what was the reason if they left school? Inquire about each parent's own parents, siblings, and the siblings' children for a similar history.

Are there any other risk factors relating to early childhood? Is there a history of abuse or neglect? Was the child in foster care? If so, why and what was the care like in this foster family?

Information relating to family history might also identify a child as at risk for academic problems. A family history of learning disabilities, including a specific type referred to as dyslexia, flags a child as at risk. Children with ADHD have a high likelihood of having a learning disability; thus if there is a family history of ADHD, the child has a likelihood of having a learning disability. Often the history is not specific. However, a parent plus possible grandparent or other close relative might have done poorly in school.

Has the family moved? If so, how did the child adjust to the move? Was there difficulty adjusting to new schools? Perhaps one school system provided a lot of supportive help, thus minimizing any school difficulties, and the new school system does not provide such help and the child is now having academic difficulties. Is there a different language spoken at home than at school?

Did the child live in a stable home environment? Are parents divorced? If so, is each family's environment stable and stress-free? What is the custody arrangement? Is either parent remarried or living with someone? Is there evidence of stress for the child because of the divorce, remarriage, or custody arrangement?

Have there been frequent moves, possibly to other states or countries? If so, how stable and consistent were the schools? How did such changes affect the child's ability to make and have friends?

## School History

The pediatrician is in a good position to be aware of the quality of the different school systems or schools attended by their patients. Perhaps specific schools or school districts are known to have minimal resources for children who need more than what the general education class can provide.

How has the child done each year of school? Has he or she struggled since preschool, or did the problems begin at a certain grade or with the change to a different school? Did the academic difficulties begin with the start of middle school or high school?

The child's school history might clarify another risk factor. If the child has struggled in school through several grades or has repeated a grade, the pediatrician must consider this possibility of a learning disability. If the child has a history of struggling with previous academic skill demands, such as reading or writing, he or she is at risk for continuing to have academic problems in later grades.

Often, adolescents are evaluated because of school-related behavioral problems. The pediatrician must consider that the frustrations and failures resulting from academic difficulties contributed to the adolescent's poor self-image and negative behaviors. An adolescent with a history of cutting classes, skipping school, or resisting or avoiding doing homework might be acting this way to cover up academic deficits, possibly a learning disability. When an adolescent is using alcohol or illegal drugs and/or is rebellious, one possible cause might be an unrecognized, or recognized but poorly treated, learning disability.

## Office-based Sources of Information

Some pediatricians ask parents to fill out a brief school performance questionnaire. Questions focus on any concerns parents might have with their child's learning or school performance as well as problems with homework. If the comments suggest difficulties, a more detailed form focused on school performance is used. If time permits, some pediatricians or other office staff might perform a screening test to identify a child's level of reading, writing, and math. There are many brief screening tests that address these issues. They are neither sensitive nor specific, but they may assist the pediatrician in delineating areas that need further exploration and evaluation by the school or by other sources.

The goal of this book is in part to provide the pediatrician with a time-efficient screening assessment model for possible learning disabilities and other related disabilities. Later chapters will go into more specific detail. The rest of this chapter will focus on our current knowledge about brain function and dysfunction as it relates to learning disabilities.

## Research on How the Brain Learns

Many years of educational, psychological, and neuropsychological research focused on neurodevelopment and the progressive maturation of the brain's capacity to learn. These studies resulted in a developmental educational model. What is the child capable of understanding and learning from birth onward? These data shaped the development of age-appropriate curricula and teaching method models. What is a child capable of learning in preschool? Kindergarten? First grade? And on? These brain developmental findings resulted in both the curricula and the best methods of teaching for each school grade.

In recent years there has been an increased demand for what are called "scientifically based teaching methods," "scientifically proven teaching materials," and "grade-specific curriculum." With the increased focus on research-based information, teacher education and continuing education programs are changing.

A major breakthrough in research relating to learning and learning disabilities occurred when it became possible to do brain imaging studies that allowed the researcher to learn how the brain processes and learns, as well as how the brain of individuals with learning disabilities might learn differently. Brain research has gone on for many years using either gross studies of brain slices or microscopic studies of areas of the brain. These were static observations of the brain and could only focus on structure. Such studies on individuals known to have dyslexia, a specific type of learning disability, clearly showed that nerve cells needed for reading were clustered closer to the surface of the cortex than they should be and that many of these nerve cells sent out connections that did not connect with another cell.

With the development of functional magnetic resonance imaging (fMRI), it became possible to study the live brain as it performed different tasks. If an individual is given a specific task, for example reading, what area(s) of the brain activates first? Next? And so on through the full process.

Does the brain process this information differently with individuals who have known learning disabilities?

Thanks to the pioneering work of Dr Sally Shaywitz and Dr Bennet Shaywitz at Yale Medical School, along with expanded research by others, using the fMRI technology we now better understand the physiology of reading and how the brains of individuals with reading disabilities process information differently than individuals without this disability. These studies are definite, showing that specific reading disabilities reflect the lack of or weaknesses in specific areas of brain function, that learning disabilities are no longer defined as "presumed to be neurologically based processing disorders" but as "neurologically based processing disorders."

Other researchers have studied other learning tasks, writing, math, organization, etc. Current research is also focused on the developmental process. How does the brain mature and at what age is the brain able to process the next level of learning needed for basic skills relating to education? (References to these researchers and their findings are listed in the Bibliography of this chapter.)

Summaries of these studies follow to illustrate basic concepts. These summaries are not meant to be comprehensive reviews of each topic or part of a topic covered. The findings help to clarify how an individual reads, writes, does math, etc. The findings also show why specific individuals might show specific learning disabilities.

## Reading

The first step in reading is to record the image (word) on the occipital cortex. The eye acts like a transducer, converting the received image into nerve impulses that relay the image to the visual cortex. Reading is a brain function. When someone connected to fMRI starts to read, it is the visual cortex that fires (lights up) first. The next area of the brain to activate is the site for auditory processing. The brain uses phonemes to process and to understand the word. Thus, for example, the word "cat" would be decoded as "k-a-t." This phonologically based code is then analyzed by areas of the cortex and interpreted to mean cat. It seems that reading requires more than decoding each word. To read "cat" does not lead to comprehension of what is read. Thus the next area of the brain to fire is related to working memory. It seems that the word "cat" is held in this transient memory site until enough words come in to allow for meaning. For example, "The cat jumped on the table." Once there is meaning, these groups of words are moved to short-term memory and this area of the brain fires. The information seems to be organized and stored. Thus the process of reading involves in sequence the visual cortex, then the auditory processing cortex, then the area of working memory, and finally the areas of short-term memory.

A child, thus, might have difficulty with recognition of letters and sounds, so critical to the first step in reading (decoding). Other children might have difficulty phonologically decoding the word to comprehend the meaning of the word. Formal testing might show difficulties with working memory or with the ability to retain (store) the information read. Later in this chapter, these steps from decoding to comprehension to memory will be discussed in more detail.

## Writing

In many ways, the process of writing is the reverse of reading. The first step is to retrieve from memory the information that will be needed to produce the desired written information. This retrieved information must be organized as needed to respond to the question or task. The relevant area of the cortex lights up. Next, clusters of information are relayed to the area of working memory. This area lights up. Next, individual words are relayed to either the area of the cortex related to motor output or to the area of the cortex related to language output. Then each phoneme in the word is relayed to the hand to produce the letter/word or to the vocal apparatus to produce the word orally.

Some individuals have difficulty finding the necessary information, retrieving this information, organizing this information, processing it through working memory, or with the ability to do the required fine motor tasks or language processing tasks. Each possible area of learning difficulty will be described later.

## Math

This area of processing is understood less. It seems that the process is similar to that required for writing. The first step is to retrieve the necessary knowledge (eg, concept, formula, equation...) as well as basic math facts (eg, times tables). These data are used to process the results needed. Next, these data are processed through working memory to the motor cortex and produced on the page. More details on possible areas of difficulty and the resulting learning problem will be discussed later.

## Organization/Executive Function

Studies show that these skills are centered in the frontal cortex. They will be described in detail later in this chapter. Specific steps and the results of something influencing these steps are not yet clear.

## *Education Developmental Model*

The curriculum and teaching methods used in the classroom have been developed based on many years of psychological and neuropsychological studies showing what the child is capable of learning at each age. The newer brain imaging studies confirm most of the basis for the models developed. Some imaging studies helped to clarify a process, leading to a change in teaching models or to changes in remedial models. A good example of this relates to reading. For many years, researchers did not always agree as to whether reading was a visual or an auditory (phonological) process. Thus one school of thought suggested teaching reading through the visual or sight recognition approach (whole words were memorized and learned). The other school of thought believed that reading was a phonological task. Early letter recognition and the ability to apply the correct phonemes to decode the word were taught. The newer fMRI studies confirm that reading is a phonological process. Thus the use of whole word recognition is used less.

Educators use knowledge of brain development to plan what can be taught at each age/grade level. Thus the educational model for teaching is a developmental model. Skills are taught in a sequential model, building on previously learned information. The basic skills of reading, writing, and math are presented first, followed by the more advanced skills relating to organization and executive function. If a child fails to acquire these basic skills in early grades, he or she will have greater challenges in later grades.

# The Basic Skills

## *Developmental Model for Reading*

In **preschool** the child needs to learn 2 basic skills. First is rapid letter recognition and second is the ability to know what sound goes with each letter. The letters are called *graphemes* and the sounds are called *phonemes*. These skills are improved during **kindergarten**.

In **first grade** the student learns to put the correct phoneme to the correct grapheme and "sound out" words. After a word has been sounded out frequently, most students recognize the whole word and can read it without the need to decode (sight reading).

In **second grade** these skills are expanded as the child learns to read faster and with greater ability to understand.

**Third grade** brings a new set of demands. The assumption is that the student can now read. The focus shifts to reading comprehension, knowing what has been read. Books are assigned and the student reads them. Gradually, through third and **fourth grade,** the length and complexity of the material read increases. This skill of reading longer and more complex content and retaining it is called *reading fluency.* By the end of fourth grade it is assumed that the student can read, comprehend, and retain what has been read.

These skills are critical because by **fifth grade and beyond** the focus shifts to using these skills to learn subject content. The subject taught (history, literature, science) becomes the primary focus.

## *Developmental Model for Writing*

In **preschool** children start to learn the letters of the alphabet and numbers (graphemes). They learn to recognize each and to form each in a specific way.

In **first grade** the child learns to write words. Gradually, he learns to write on a line and to have a space between words. Later he learns to capitalize the first word and to put a period at the end. During first and then **second grade,** the ability to write becomes easier and more fluid. Initially spelling might be "creative," but soon correct spelling is expected.

By **third grade** it is assumed that the student can write with basic spelling, capitalization, and punctuation. Grammar skills are improved, as well as the student's ability to get his or her thoughts organized and onto the page. The focus shifts from "can you write" to a greater focus on "what have you written." The student starts to do book reports and journals. If a child has difficulty with handwriting, it will become an issue in third grade. (This grapho-motor problem will be discussed in Chapter 5.) These skills are expanded and improved in **fourth grade.**

By **fifth grade**, the assumption is that basic writing skills are in place. As with reading, the focus shifts to learning subject content. The ability to write with correct spelling, grammar, punctuation, and capitalization is expected. (These 4 skills are often called *language arts skills*.) Book reports and journal entries expand into writing stories and longer answers to questions. This skill of flowing thoughts onto the page is called *writing fluency*. This focus on content continues with increasing demands through **middle** and **high school.**

## Developmental Model for Math

In **preschool and kindergarten** the child learns to recognize numbers and starts to learn to count. In **first and second grades** 2 basic concepts are taught. First is the concept of "base 10." Our number system is based on units of 10. The second concept is referred to as the "conservation of numbers." Numbers cannot be created or eliminated. The child learns to put numbers together and to take numbers away (addition and subtraction). In **third grade**, these learned skills are used to teach multiplication and division. **Fourth grade and fifth grade** are used to consolidate these skills. Layers of increased math knowledge are added (fractions, decimals, and more).

These basic skills are essential for the child to learn advanced math in **middle and high school** (eg, algebra, geometry, calculus). Each year builds on knowledge learned in previous years.

# *The Higher-Level Skills*

## Organization

Organizational skills are introduced and taught in **first through fifth grades.** Gradually, the student learns to organize notebooks, backpacks, and papers as well as to keep track of assignments and when assignments are due. Slowly, teachers pull back and expect the student to have these skills and to use them on their own. By **middle school** such skills are expected. In **high school** they are critical.

It is important to understand the specifics about organizational skills. These skills include the ability to organize materials as well as to organize information. Keeping track of notebooks, papers, and other school materials is essential. Yet it is also necessary to organize information into small units and then larger units in order to process, store, and later retrieve information. Each aspect of organization is critical.

### Developmental Model for Organizing Materials

In **preschool and early elementary school** teachers introduce the concepts of organization of materials. Where is your cubicle or shelf? What goes there? What do you need for each activity? What goes home and what needs to come back? These procedures are practiced. Parents learn what should be in the backpack when the child comes home and what should be in it when she returns to school. If the child has difficulties with these skills, supports are provided.

In the **fourth and fifth grades** these support systems are slowly removed and the child is expected to know what goes where, what to bring to class, class routines, what goes home, and what is to come back. Now losing, forgetting, and misplacing papers and projects becomes an issue. Homework must be done, taken to school, and turned in.

This need for organizing materials is critical in **middle school.** The child now has 6 or more teachers, each with a different teaching style, way of using materials, and expectations. What papers and worksheets go in which folder or binder? Where does he put his homework so that he will find it to turn in during class? The student must keep track of 5 or more homework assignments, knowing what must go home, what must come back, when it is due, and where to put it on each teacher's desk. The middle school curriculum in most school systems recognizes this increased demand for organizational skills. Thus in sixth grade, there is often a "safety net." Teachers remind students what their assignments are and what they will need to take home. Parents are often instructed to help with the return process. Teachers often remind students to turn in their homework. Gradually, this safety net is removed and the student is expected to organize without reminders. If a student is having difficulty keeping track of assignments, papers, and other materials, the teacher might give extra help.

By **high school** it is assumed that the student has full organizational skills and can function independently. Homework and other assignments are expected to be turned in on time with no reminders. Deadlines are to be met.

### Developmental Model for Organizing Information

By **middle school** it is important that the student learns to organize the information read. Rote memory is not as effective in learning as storing what is learned in clumps or units of information that can be understood. The more organized the information, the easier it is to study and to learn. Writing demands become longer and more complex. The student needs to retrieve information and then organize this information before starting to write. Before a math problem can be done, it is necessary to retrieve the necessary math facts and equations and organize this information in the proper order before starting to write the calculations and answers.

The amount of material that must be organized and learned increases through **high school.** Writing assignments become more complex, requiring a greater degree of organization of learned material. (Example, "Give four reasons for the collapse of the Roman Empire and use examples to document each.")

### Executive Function

As tasks become more complex, it is important to be able to analyze the task, lay out a plan of action, monitor these efforts, and complete the task in a timely way. This process is referred to as executive function and is located in the prefrontal cortex. Increased maturation of this area of the brain in early adolescents significantly increases the student's executive function skills. For this reason, increasing demand for these abilities is introduced in **middle school** and expected by **high school.**

What is the assignment? What needs to be done? How will it be approached and in what order? What timelines must be met to have a completed assignment ready to turn in on time? With this plan, what do I have to do during this day? Tomorrow? The weekend?

In **middle school** teachers illustrate and teach these skills. The class is given a written assignment. The teacher helps the class set up an outline and establish timelines. The class works as a group, completing each step and presenting it for discussion and editing, then presents a finished product. By **high school** it is assumed that students can carry out these executive functions independently. For a summary of the stages of learning, see Boxes 2.1 through 2.6.

---

### Box 2-1. Learning to Read

*Preschool/Kindergarten*
- Rapid letter recognition
- Phonics

*First/Second Grades*
- Learn to read.

*Third/Fourth Grades*
- Learn reading comprehension.

*Fifth Grade*
- Increasing ability to read longer and more complex material and retain what is read (reading fluency)

*Middle School*
- Shift from reading as a skill to reading as a way to learn content.

*High School*
- Reading fluency is assumed. The focus is only on content.

## Box 2-2. Learning to Write

*Preschool/Kindergarten*
- Develop motor skills.
- Learn to form letters correctly.

*First/Second Grades*
- Learn to form letters correctly, on line, and in correct place.
- Learn capitalization and early punctuation.
- Early spelling

*Third/Fourth Grades*
- Learn spelling, grammar, punctuation, and capitalization (language arts).
- Learn to organize content.

*Fifth Grade*
- Learn to organize thoughts and to write full and complete answers and reports.

*Middle/High School*
- Increasingly learn to organize and to write longer and more complex answers and reports.

## Box 2-3. Learning to Do Math

*Preschool/Kindergarten*
- Learn to recognize and to form numbers.

*First/Second Grades*
- Learn the concept of "base 10."
- Learn the concept of "conservation of numbers," leading to learning addition and subtraction.

*Third/Fourth/Fifth Grades*
- Learn multiplication and division.
- Learn fractions, decimals, and more.

*Middle/High School*
- Apply learned knowledge to progressively learn higher-level math.

## Box 2-4. Learning Organizational Skills

*Early Elementary School*
- Learn basic routines.
- Learn basic organizational skills.

*Later Elementary School*
- Learn more complex routines.
- Learn more complex organizational skills.

*Middle School*
- Learn to organize what is read (reading fluency).
- Learn to organize what is to be written (writing fluency).
- Learn to organize previously learned and new information and apply to doing math calculations (math fluency).
- Learn to organize information into meaningful clusters in order to learn.

*High School*
- Increasingly master greater demands of reading, writing, and math fluency.

## Box 2-5. Executive Function Skills

*Middle School*
- Learn strategies for learning and time planning.

*High School*
- Develop increasingly more complex ability to analyze, develop, and carry out learning tasks with effective strategies.
- Develop increasing ability for time planning and completing tasks in a timely way.

---

## Box 2-6. Summary of Learning Skills

*Reading*
- Learn to read.
- Reading comprehension
- Reading fluency

*Writing*
- Learn to write.
- Learn language arts skills.
- Writing fluency

*Math*
- Learn basic facts.
- Apply basics to learn advanced facts.
- Math fluency

*Organization*
- Learn basic routines.
- Learn to organize materials.
- Learn to organize concepts, flow of thoughts.
- Learn to organize information to be learned and to be written.

*Executive Function*
- Learn strategies for doing tasks.
- Learn time planning.

---

In Chapter 3 this developmental model of education will be used to develop an educational review of systems. Positive findings from this review would suggest possible learning disabilities.

# *Bibliography*

Denckla MB. Executive function: binding together the definitions of attention-deficit/hyperactivity disorder and learning disabilities. In: Lynn Meltzer, ed. *Executive Function in Education. From Theory to Practice*. New York, NY: Guilford Press; 2007:5–18

Kelly DP, Aylward GP. Identifying school performance problems in the pediatric office. *Pediatr Ann.* 2005;34(4):288–298

Lambros KM, Leslie LK. Management of the child with a learning disorder. *Pediatr Ann.* 2005;34(4):275–287

Lerner J, Kline F. *Learning Disabilities and Related Disorders. Characteristics and Teaching Strategies*. 10th ed. New York, NY: Houghton Mifflin Co.; 2006

Lyon GR, Rumsey JM, eds. *Neuroimaging. A Window to the Neurological Foundations of Learning and Behavior in Children.* Baltimore, MD: Brookes; 2006

Miller KJ. Executive functions. *Pediatr Ann.* 2005;34(4):310–317

Shaywitz S. *Overcoming Dyslexia. A New and Complete Science-Based Program for Reading Problems at Any Level.* New York, NY: Alfred A. Knopf; 2003

Shaywitz SE, Shaywitz BA, Pugh KR, et al. The neurobiology of developmental dyslexia as viewed through the lens of functional magnetic resonance imaging technology. In: Lyon GR, Rumsey JM, eds. *Neuroimaging. A Window to the Neurological Foundations of Learning and Behavior in Children.* Baltimore, MD: Brookes; 2006:57–78

# Chapter 3

*Diagnosing Learning Disabilities*

Learning disabilities are caused by neurologically based processing disorders. These "wiring" problems are at the cellular level and are not detectable on neurologic assessments or studies (eg, electroencephalograms, brain scans). These processing deficits were first recognized through neuropsychological studies and now have been validated by brain imaging studies. Functional magnetic resonance imaging of normal children shows the areas of the brain that activate and in what sequence during each phase of doing specific academic tasks. Similar studies of children with learning disabilities clearly show where this process is interrupted, resulting in dysfunctional processing and causing the disability. Educational research shows that in the area of reading, early interventions using a phonics-based method leads to changes within the brain, suggesting that the brain may be able to correct or compensate for initial deficits. Although preliminary, these findings add more importance to early recognition, diagnosis, and intervention. Let's say a child comes into the office with a sore throat and fever. Physical examination reveals enlarged cervical lymph nodes and tonsils with exudate. A diagnosis is suspected but not finalized. Further studies are done, probably including a rapid strep test and maybe a throat culture, monospot, or complete blood count. If the laboratory studies confirm the initial clinical impression, appropriate treatment is started. The same clinical model is used in diagnosing a learning disability. The history suggests such a possibility. An educational review of systems either rules out or further supports your clinical impression. Your clinical impression is confirmed by formal testing (to be discussed in Chapter 8). Once confirmed, a medical treatment plan can be initiated. This review of systems is based on knowing what questions to ask in order to clarify if the child or adolescent might have problems with academic skills (reading, writing, math, organization, executive function) or with language or motor skills. The data collected are compared with where the patient should be for his or her age and grade. The results help focus the types of further testing needed. Keep in mind the developmental model discussed in Chapter 2 (Box 3-1).

---

**Box 3-1. Skills Expected to Be Mastered at Particular Grade Levels**

| | |
|---|---|
| Preschool/Kindergarten: | Introduction to pre-academic skills |
| First/Second Grades: | Learn basic skills of reading, writing, math. |
| Third/Fourth Grades: | Learn to use these skills. |
| Fifth/Middle School: | Skills are assumed; focus is on content. Learn to use organization/executive function skills. |
| High School: | Focus is totally on content; skills assumed; organization and executive function skills are essential. |

This model leads to the questions you might ask based on the age and grade of the patient.

---

## Review of Systems for Learning Disabilities

A reproducible worksheet with the following questions can be found in Appendix B.

### Preschool/Kindergarten

Reading:    "Can your child recognize letters and numbers?"

Writing:    "Does your child have difficulties with coloring or cutting? Is your child learning to form letters and numbers?"

Math:       "Is your child learning the meaning of numbers? Is your child able to count to 10? 20? 30?"

### First/Second Grade

Reading:    "Can your child sound out words? Does your child recognize words learned earlier? Is your child reading at the level of the other children?"

Writing:    "Can your child form all letters and numbers? Does your child write on the line? Capitalize? Punctuate?"

Math:       "Has your child mastered addition? Subtraction?"

### Third/Fourth Grade

Reading: "Does your child understand what he or she reads? Does your child enjoy reading?"

Writing: "Has your child learned to capitalize? Punctuate? Does your child spell as well as the teacher expects? Can your child write full sentences that respond to the teacher's request?"

Math: "Can your child do multiplication? Division? Is your child at the level of skills expected by the teacher?"

### Fifth and Above

Reading: "Can your child read with ease and understand what is read? Does your child retain the information from reading?"

Writing: "Can your child organize thoughts and get them down on the page? Are your child's answers to questions and assignments seen as complete and fully addressing the material?"

Math: "Are your child's math skills at the level expected by the teacher for his or her grade? Can your child do calculations without making too many careless errors?"

Organization: "Are your child's papers, notebooks, binders, and backpack neat and organized? Does your child lose, forget, or misplace papers and other materials? What about your child's desk? Locker? Bedroom? Does your child have difficulty organizing facts to learn or to write?"

Executive Function: "Is your child good at planning out how to do homework? Does your child get work done on time?"

## Case Examples Using the Educational Review of Systems

Let's go back to Alex, the 10-year-old boy mentioned in Chapter 2. Initial screening suggested that, although he is misbehaving, he did not have attention-deficit/hyperactivity disorder (ADHD), nor did he seem to have a primary emotional problem. You start your assessment for a possible learning disability. Alex is in the fifth grade, so you know what skills would be expected of him for this grade. Your questions are focused on clarifying if he has these skills. Getting clear answers from children is not always easy. Thus you might word your questions in a way that assists the child to focus on what you need to know. You start with reading:

*Dr Smith:* "Alex, is reading something you like to do or that you have to do?"

*Alex:* "I only read when I have to. I like to read sports magazines only."

*Dr Smith:* "What happens when you have to read school papers or books?"

*Alex:* "I mess up and forget."

*Dr Smith:* "Help me understand this problem. For example, is your problem with sounding out or understanding the words?"

*Alex:* "No."

*Dr Smith:* "Do you find that sometimes you can read and understand what you are reading, but when you get to the end, you forgot what you have read so you cannot answer the questions without having to go back and find the answers?"

*Alex:* "Yes, all the time."

*Dr Smith:* "Alex, do you sometimes get papers back and realize that you misread the questions or instructions?"

*Alex:* "How did you know? I do this all of the time."

At this point, you suspect that he can read and comprehend, but Alex might have problems with reading fluency, a skill required in fifth grade.

Next, you go to writing:

*Dr Smith:* "How would you describe your handwriting?"

*Alex:* "It is messy unless I go slow. But if I go slow I don't finish, so I write fast and the teacher complains that she cannot read it."

*Dr Smith:* "Can you write fast enough to copy from the board or overhead or write down assignments?"

*Alex:* "Yes, I write fast, but I can't read my own handwriting."

*Dr Smith:* "When you look at what you wrote, do you find any problems with spelling?"

*Alex:* "I can't spell."

*Dr Smith:* "How about grammar, punctuation, or capitalization?"

*Alex:* "I'm horrible at them."

*Dr Smith:* "When you have to write an answer, a report, or a paper, do you ever have problems getting your thoughts together in your head and then writing them on the page?"

*Alex:* "My teacher always complains that I do not write enough or that what I write does not always fit together."

You now suspect a problem with language arts—spelling, grammar, punctuation, capitalization—as well as with writing fluency. You also wonder if he might have a grapho-motor problem.

Now, you move on to math.

*Dr Smith:* "Do you feel that you know all of the math facts that you are expected to know in class?"

*Alex:* "I'm not too good at long division and keep forgetting my times tables."

*Dr Smith:* "You must have a hard time doing the math expected for fifth grade."

*Alex:* "I stink at math. My dad has to help me do my homework every night."

*Dr Smith:* "Do you ever misread the word problem or instructions and then answer incorrectly?"

*Alex:* "Yes."

*Dr Smith:* "Do you get papers back and find that you made careless errors—adding when you meant to subtract, multiplying wrong, skipping steps, leaving out part of the problem?"

*Alex:* "You must have seen my papers. I think I know what to do, but I make stupid mistakes. I wish I could just do it in my head and write down the answer, but my teacher won't let me."

You suspect weakness in basic math skills as well as errors because of his possible reading fluency. You also suspect a math fluency problem.

Now, on to organization and executive function—skills increasingly in demand in fifth grade.

*Dr Smith:* "Alex, I am almost finished. Thanks for being so helpful. What do your notebook, binders, and backpack look like? Do you sometimes lose or forget things?"

*Alex:* "Did my mom tell you? Everything is a mess. I always lose things or put them in the wrong place and then not find them."

*Dr Smith:* "Do you ever get to school and realize that you left something at home. Or, do you get home from school and realize that you left something in school?"

*Alex:* "Yep."

*Dr Smith:* "How about your desk, locker, and bedroom?"

*Alex:* "They are the same, a mess."

*Dr Smith:* "You told me earlier that you have difficulty when you have to write an answer or a paper. Do you think the problem might be that you also have a problem organizing your thoughts so that you know what to write?"

*Alex:* "Yea. But, if mom discusses what I am going to write first, it is OK."

*Dr Smith:* "When you have to learn something, is it easy or hard to get all of the information together so that it makes sense and you can learn it?"

*Alex:* "If the teacher asks a specific question I am OK, but if I have to answer a bigger question, like tell about something in a book we read, I have trouble."

*Dr Smith:* "Can you keep track of time and get your work done on time and turned in on time?"

*Alex:* "I'm always late or forget."

You now add to your list the possibility of an organization and executive function problem.

*Dr Smith:* "You know, Alex, it sounds like school is hard for you and that you are trying your best but not doing well. No wonder you are frustrated and angry in school. We need to find out why and then find ways to help you. I am going to talk to your parents about having some studies done to help me better understand why someone as bright as you is struggling in school. Then I will work with your school to get you the help you need. Is this OK with you?"

*Alex:* "Fine, thanks."

This educational review of systems took about 5 to 10 minutes to do. You now have a clinical impression and can move on to rule this impression in or rule it out. Chapter 9 will discuss how such studies are done.

## Conclusion

The critical first step in diagnosing a learning disability is recognizing that such a possibility exists. Based on the information provided by the parents and the information collected from the educational review of systems, the possibility that the school problems are related to a learning disability will become clear. Formal studies can then be requested resulting in confirming the diagnosis. The diagnostic process is no different than getting a clinical history of a sore throat and observing enlarged cervical lymph nodes and tonsils with exudate, then ordering specific laboratory studies. The chief complaint leads to more detailed information on present illness and history, the physical examination leads to any necessary diagnostic studies, and the final results lead to a diagnosis and a medical treatment plan. The focus of this chapter has been on learning disabilities. This focus is not to minimize the need to explore for other school-based problems (eg, substandard schools, or cultural or bilingual problems). There might also be family dynamics or other social issues that explain or contribute to the academic difficulties. Is school success a high priority with the family? As will be discussed in Chapter 8, about 50% of children with learning disabilities will also have ADHD. Often the diagnosis of ADHD is made first, the disorder is treated, and the child can now to sit and focus. However, it becomes clearer that there are academic problems above those caused by the ADHD. The medications will be continued; however, the focus now shifts to clarifying if there might be a learning disability.

# Chapter 4

# The Related Language Disabilities

It is not uncommon for children with learning disabilities to also have a language disability. Thus it is important to screen for these disabilities as well.

A speech and/or language delay will have a significant effect on personal, social, academic, and future vocational life. Although some children will develop normal speech and language skills without treatment by the time they enter school, it is essential to identify those who will not.

Some references for parents suggest that speech-language interventions should not begin until the child begins to talk. This advice is incorrect. Studies show that children know a great deal about their language even before the first word is said. As examples, infants and toddlers can distinguish between their native language and a foreign language, use different nonverbal utterances to express different needs, and imitate different patterns of speech through babbling.

Children identified as at risk or high risk, such as those who spend time in neonatal intensive care units, should be tested early and at regular intervals. Other risk factors include diagnosed medical conditions, such as chronic ear infections or lead poisoning; biological factors, such as fetal alcohol syndrome; genetic defects, such as Down syndrome; neurologic defects, such as cerebral palsy; or a family history of language disorders. Children with no obvious high risk factors should be evaluated if their speech and language are not similar to those of other children of the same age.

Early intervention services are available through federal mandate in every community to provide such evaluations and treatment services. More details on these federal mandates are in Chapter 10.

# Normal Language Milestones

Literature from speech and language professionals offers general guidelines for language development and specific milestones and clinical clues of a possible problem. The general guidelines focus on the overall clarity of the child's speech, or intelligibility. A commonly used guide for a general assessment of development is referred to as the rule of fourths.

- By 18 months of age, the average toddler's speech is understandable to strangers *one-fourth* of the time but is clear to the mother 95% of the time.
- By 2 years of age, someone who sees the child often probably understands him *half* of the time while his parents understand him 98% of the time.
- By 3 years of age, the average child's speech is expected to be comprehensible to strangers *three-fourths* of the time while being clear to close family members 100% of the time.
- By the time the child is 4 years old, her speech is completely understandable *all* of the time to all listeners.

Specific guidelines are important to consider during well-child checks. Each noted area of difficulty might suggest a clinical clue and the need for further assessments. Listed below are specific guidelines collated from several standard checklists developed by speech and language professionals. Normal language milestones are noted for specific age periods. Causes for concern for each age period are noted in Box 4-1.

# Language Disabilities

A language processing problem might involve the ability to receive auditory information (receptive language) or the ability to organize and retrieve thoughts and express them orally (expressive language). Children with a language disability might have a receptive disability, an expressive disability, or both.

As noted in Chapter 1, in the *Diagnostic and Statistical Manual of Mental Disorders, Fourth Edition, Text Revision* these difficulties are called *language disorders.* Three subtypes are listed: receptive language disorder, expressive language disorder, and mixed receptive-expressive language disorders. Within the fields of education and special education and within the field of speech and language therapy, the same 3 types of problems are noted.

## Box 4-1. Language Milestones by Age Group

### First 3 Months

**Expected Behaviors**
- Looks at caregivers/others
- Becomes quiet in response to sound
- Smiles or coos in response to voice
- Cries differently when tired, hungry, in pain

**Cause for Concern**
- Lack of responsiveness
- Lack of awareness of sound
- Lack of awareness of environment
- Cry is no different if tired, hungry, in pain
- Problems suckling/swallowing

### 3 to 6 Months

**Expected Behaviors**
- Fixes gaze on face
- Responds to name by looking at source of voice
- Identifies location of sound
- Cooing, gurgling, chuckling, laughing

**Cause for Concern**
- Cannot focus
- Lack of awareness of sound; not looking toward source
- Lack of awareness of people, objects

### 6 to 9 Months

**Expected Behaviors**
- Imitates vocalizing
- Enjoys social interaction games by adults (peek-a-boo, pat-a-cake)
- Has different vocalizations for different emotional states
- Babbling, vocal play with sounds
- Cries when parent leaves room
- Responds to soft speech and environmental sounds

**Cause for Concern**
- Does not appear to understand or enjoy the social rewards of interaction
- Lack of connection with adults (lack of eye contact, reciprocal eye gaze)
- No babbling or minimal babbling

### 9 to 12 Months

**Expected Behaviors**
- Attracts attention (vocalizing, coughing)
- Shakes head no, pushes some objects away
- Waves good-bye
- Indicates requests clearly (pats or pulls adult and points to object)
- Imitates new sounds/actions
- Shows consistent patterns of sounds that sound like first words ("ma-ma," "da-da")

**Cause for Concern**
- Easily upset by sounds that do not upset others
- May look at object but not indicate he wants it
- Lack of responses indicating comprehension of words or gestures

### 12 to 18 Months

**Expected Behaviors**
- Single-word speech begins
- Requests objects by pointing, vocalizing
- Gets attention vocally ("mommy")
- Uses ritual words ("bye," "hi," "please")
- Protests: "no," shakes head, moves away
- Acknowledges: eye contact, vocal response

**Cause for Concern**
- Does not attempt to imitate or produce words to convey meaning
- Does not persist in verbal request
- Limited comprehension (fewer than 15 words or phrases to communicate) by 18 months
- Limited expressive vocabulary using fewer than 15 words by 18 months

## Box 4-1. Language Milestones by Age Group, continued

### 18 to 24 Months

**Expected Behaviors**
- Uses mostly words to communicate
- Begins to use 2-word combinations ("daddy car" when father leaves)
- By 24 months has at least 50 words

**Cause for Concern**
- Reliance on gestures without words
- Limited expressive vocabulary
- Does not use 2-word combinations by 24 months
- Largely unintelligible speech by 24 months

### 24 to 36 Months

**Expected Behaviors**
- Engages in short dialogues
- Talks when playing alone
- Expresses emotions
- Uses language in imaginary ways
- Uses attention-getting devices ("hey")
- Begins to include the articles (a, the) and word endings (-ing, -s)
- Understands simple 2-step commands

**Cause for Concern**
- Words limited to single syllables
- Few or no multi-word utterances
- Does not demand response from listener
- Asks no questions
- Poor speech intelligibility
- Tantrums when not understood
- May echo or parrot words
- Unable to comprehend language unless spoken simply and slowly

### 36 to 48 Months

**Expected Behaviors**
- Begins to learn from listening
- Carries on conversation
- Asks questions (who? how?)
- Uses pronouns correctly
- Uses language to create pretend situations

**Cause for Concern**
- Frequently says "huh?" or needs directions repeated
- Limited vocabulary
- Frustrated in communicative situations
- Substitutes me/I, him/he, her/she
- Little language during pretend play

### 48 to 60 Months

**Expected Behaviors**
- Can explain how an object is used
- Can talk about past, future, and imaginary events
- People outside the family understand him

**Cause for Concern**
- Difficulty with word finding when asked to explain how objects are used
- Unable to retell stories or recent events
- Sentences seem unorganized and loose
- Only family members understand him

However, the term *disability* is used rather than disorder. When communicating with health insurance companies, the term *language disorder* must be used. When interacting with school systems, the term *language disability* will be more appropriate.

# Receptive Language Disability

The neurologic processes involved in receiving and processing sounds are similar in most ways to the steps involved in receiving and processing visual stimuli, such as when reading. Specifically, auditory perception includes
- Sound localization and lateralization
- Recording the sound inputs as quickly as they are received
- Decoding the words received
- Recording these words in working memory
- Recording these words in short-term memory

Some professionals expand the tasks involved in auditory perception and refer to this broader concept as *central auditory processing*. The focus is on the individual's ability to process sound input when there might be competing acoustic signals or when the auditory signals are unclear. That is, how does one interpret auditory information when it is presented in a less than optimal listening environment? There is no general agreement on the definition, what test should be used, and how to interpret these results.

A receptive language disability might involve one or more of the steps described above. A child must recognize where a sound is coming from. He is on the playground and hears a friend call his name. Is the sound coming from the left or right? In front or behind? The ability to localize the source of the sound and perhaps look in that direction is important. Difficulty with this process of lateralization is often called an *auditory figure-ground* problem. A parent might recognize this problem and call the child's name, requesting eye contact before speaking, saying "Look at me."

Next, the child must record the sounds received as quickly as they come in. Some children have difficulty processing sound inputs as quickly as the rate of normal speech. This difficulty is often called an *auditory lag*. The person is speaking at a normal rate, yet the child cannot receive and process the sounds at that speed. Some parents intuitively learn this and find that they need to speak slower to their child, giving one instruction at a time.

Once the sounds are received and recorded, the child must be able to distinguish the subtle differences in sounds (phonemes), much as reading required distinguishing subtle differences in shapes (graphemes). Once decoded, the child must analyze and understand what each word means. Each word is then floated in working memory until they blend into a meaningful concept. This cluster of words (concept) is then moved to short-term memory.

Thus children with a receptive language disability might have difficulties in one or more of the following areas:

- Auditory lateralization (auditory figure-ground)
- Speed of auditory processing (auditory lag)
- Auditory analysis
- Auditory working memory
- Auditory short-term memory

Receptive language difficulties can easily be misunderstood as the child not paying attention. One of the authors (LBS) remembers observing a first-grade boy because the teacher thought he had an attentional problem and might need medication. The class was busy working at their desks. This boy was drawing a picture to illustrate the story the teacher just read to the class. The teacher suddenly said, "Children, it is time for recess. Put your things away in your desk, go get your coats, and line up at the door." All of the other children followed these oral instructions. The boy being observed looked up and appeared to be confused. He watched what the other children were doing and followed what they did (put things away, get coats, go to door). The teacher then commented, "See what I mean. He was daydreaming and not paying attention." The teacher might have been correct; however, follow-up assessments showed that he had a receptive language disability. He was not able to analyze and process the teacher's request at the same rate as the other children.

## Expressive Language Disability

The steps involved in expressing oneself with words are similar to the steps involved in expressing oneself in writing. First, the child must retrieve from memory the information and words needed to speak. The next steps involve moving these thoughts into working memory, decoding the words, and relaying the pattern of phonemes to the vocal systems in order to produce the words. And the words must flow at a correct rate and rhythm. If the child initiates the conversation (spontaneous language), the thoughts might flow from memory quickly; however, if the child must respond to a situation by finding the information needed, organizing this information, and finding the right words to use (demand language), he or she might struggle to organize what to say and to find the right words. Thus expressive language disabilities might involve

- Retrieving the necessary facts
- Organizing these facts
- Selecting the correct words to use
- Passing this information into working memory
- Coding the words into their phonemes
- Relaying these phonemes to the vocal systems (larynx, oral and nasal chambers, tongue and lips)

Children with an expressive language disability might have little difficulty if they initiate the conversation. The child starts to talk about something that happened in school and chatters away. However, when asked a question or asked to respond to information, the same child might struggle to organize her thoughts and find the right words to use. Often this child gets frustrated and says, "Oh, forget it." or "I don't know." She might respond to an oral request with, "huh?" or "what?"

## *Mixed Receptive-Expressive Language Disability*

Children who are unable to analyze and process language or respond to information are diagnosed as having mixed receptive-expressive language disability. The characteristics found are a blend of the problems described previously for each.

## *What About Pragmatic Language?*

Pragmatic language refers to the ability to process, interpret, and respond to social language. Can the child read visual or auditory clues that suggest how the other person is feeling or is responding to him? Does she understand how her body language is understood by others? This aspect of language is not part of the concepts of receptive and/or expressive language disabilities, but may also be a problem for a child. It will be discussed as part of Chapter 9.

## A Review of Systems Model for Assessing for a Language Disability

**A reproducible worksheet with the following questions can be found in Appendix B.**

### With Parents

Start by exploring for a receptive language disability.

> "Do you find that it helps to get eye contact when you speak to your child?"

> "Can you give more than one instruction at a time and the child retains it?"

> "Do teachers say that your child does not seem to be paying attention to oral instructions in class?"

If the child has a receptive language problem, the parent will smile and go beyond a yes or no answer. "I always need eye contact. I have to put my hands on his cheeks and say, 'Look at me' before I speak." Or, a parent might add, "I can only give her one instruction at a time. Even two and she forgets the second. I give one, wait until it is done, then give the next." Often, the child who is unable to process receptive language is seen as inattentive and referred for an evaluation of possible attention-deficit/hyperactivity disorder (ADHD).

Next, explore for an expressive language disability.

> "When your child starts to talk to you, does he have any problems expressing himself?"

> "What happens when you ask her a question and she has to answer? Does she have any difficulty finding the words needed and expressing herself?"

Again, if there is an expressive language problem, parents will immediately pick up on the questions and describe if there are problems. You might hear, "When he starts to tell me something, he can go on and on. It is hard to get him to stop. But, when I ask him something, he might ignore me or start to answer and then ramble all over the place. Finally, he says, 'forget it' or 'I forgot' and stops."

### With the Child

The possibility of a language disability may already be suspected based on your interactions with the child during your evaluation and examination. She might be speaking and/or responding slower or it is harder to get her to focus on what you ask. It might have been hard to get a conversation started. Or, she might answer all questions with, "I don't know."

Start questions exploring for a receptive language disability.

> "When the teacher is speaking to the class, do you sometimes have trouble understanding or keeping up with what is being said?"

> "Do you sometimes find that you don't understand what people are saying and then give the wrong answer?"

> "When people are talking, do you find that you have to concentrate so hard on what they are saying that you sometimes fall behind and miss everything being said?"

> "If the teacher talks too much, do you get lost, not remembering what is being said?"

Next, ask questions exploring for an expressive language disability.

> "Do you sometimes have trouble getting your thoughts together when you have to answer a question?"

> "Do you sometimes find that you can't find the word you want to use when you are talking?"

> "I noticed that when you told me about your vacation, you had a lot to say and had no problem telling me all about it. But when I asked you a question about something else, you seemed not to know what to say and said, 'I don't know.' Do you have the same problems at home? In school? With friends?"

## Speech-Language Evaluation and Treatment

If a speech or language problem is suspected, a formal evaluation by a speech and language therapist will be needed. This assessment usually includes a combination of standardized tests, direct observation in the classroom and with parents, and analysis of observed speech samples.

These studies might be done by someone in private practice or by someone within the public school system. Testing for a hearing loss is always an essential part of the assessment. Thus, when indicated, an audiologist or otolaryngologists might be needed.

Treatment is usually done by a speech and language therapist along with modifications within the classroom. The type, frequency of visits, and length of treatment depends on the diagnoses and the rate of progress.

## Conclusion

A language disability is a significant problem in school, within the family, and in social interactions. It is important to recognize clinical clues suggesting a language delay or a possible language disability. The earliest clues should become apparent during well-child checks.

As with a learning disability, a language disability might not become apparent until the diagnosis of ADHD is established and medication started. Only then will the difficulties receiving or expressing language become apparent. It is also possible that what was thought to be inattention was a reflection of a language disability.

## Bibliography

Again MC, Geng LF, Nicholl MJ. *The Late Talker. What to Do If Your Child Isn't Talking Yet.* New York, NY: St Martin's Press; 2003

American Psychiatric Association. *Diagnostic and Statistical Manual of Mental Disorders.* 4th ed. Text rev. Washington, DC: American Psychiatric Association; 1994

Schum RL. Language screening in the pediatric office setting. *Pediatr Clin North Am.* 2007;54(3):425–436

# Chapter 5

# The Related Motor Disabilities

Children with learning disabilities might also have problems with motor skills. In the *Diagnostic and Statistical Manual of Mental Disorders, Fourth Edition (DSM-IV)* only one such disorder is identified: developmental coordination disorder. This disorder most frequently presents as a handwriting problem, sometimes referred to as a *grapho-motor disability*. This disorder will be discussed first.

## The DSM-IV Definition

As noted initially in this chapter, in *DSM-IV-TR,* motor disabilities are called *developmental coordination disorders*. As described in Chapter 1, this disorder is defined as

A. Performance in daily activities that require motor or coordination is substantially below that expected given the person's chronological age and measured intelligence. This may be manifested by marked delays in achieving motor milestones (eg, walking, crawling, sitting), dropping things, "clumsiness," poor performance in sports or poor handwriting.

B. The disturbance in Criterion A significantly interferes with academic achievement or activities of daily living.

C. The disturbance is not due to a general medical condition (eg, cerebral palsy, hemiplegia, or muscular dystrophy) and does not meet criteria for a pervasive developmental disorder.

D. If mental retardation is present, the motor difficulties are in excess of those usually associated with it.

## Sensory Processing Disorder

This fine motor problem might explain difficulty with handwriting, but the pediatrician might also hear that this child has evidence of other fine motor problems. They might have difficulty with such visual-motor tasks as catching, hitting, or throwing a ball. Or they might have difficulty with visual-spatial tasks and bump into things or knock things over.

The pediatrician may see children who have more than a fine motor problem. They appear to have difficulty with age-appropriate gross motor skills such as walking or running. Some may have weak upper trunk muscles causing them to fatigue easily when upright.

Parents of such children might complain that their child is very sensitive to touch. He does not like the tag on his shirt. She does not like the elastic in her underwear. Socks are worn inside out because the seam bothers their feet. These same parents might say that their child does not like to be held and complains when touched.

Sometimes these expanded motor-related difficulties are found with children within the pervasive developmental disorder spectrum, from autism to asperger's disorder. Other children will show no clinical evidence to suggest a pervasive developmental disorder but might show a developmental coordination disorder, possibly with clinical evidence of a learning and/or language disability.

The earliest efforts to understand children with these patterns of sensory-motor difficulties were developed by A. Jean Ayres in the 1960s. She termed her concepts *sensory integration.* Individuals with difficulties in these areas were referred to as having a *sensory integration disorder.* She believed that difficulties with sensory inputs such as gravitational, tactile, proprioceptive, vestibular, visual, and auditory sensations would result in difficulty establishing such complex skills as language, emotional regulation, and computation.

Within the past 10 or more years, researchers such as Miller and her colleagues developed a new schema than that initially developed by Ayres, proposing a new classification system. These models are referred to as a *sensory processing disorder* (SPD). At this time there is no established standardized diagnostic system or specific therapeutic interventions for each aspect of an SPD. For these reasons, the American Academy of Pediatrics (AAP) Committee on Children With Disabilities published its concerns about prescribing SPD-related therapy services for children with motor disabilities. Many of these concerns relate to SPD as an intervention for children within the pervasive developmental disorder spectrum. However, similar concerns are expressed about using SPD as an intervention for children with learning disabilities or developmental coordination disorder.

The concerns the AAP has with the current status of the understanding of SPD, how it is diagnosed, and what treatments are prescribed are valid at this time. However, because these concepts are practiced by many occupational therapists and, thus, a pediatrician's patient might be receiving such treatments, the authors believe that the pediatrician should be familiar with this concept and with this approach; thus it will be presented as Miller and her colleagues describe it.

This expanded view of sensory integration focuses on the relationship between neurologic processes such as sensory inputs and motor outputs on daily life skills, sensory-motor abilities, and behavioral difficulties. As explained earlier in this chapter, although not yet accepted by the AAP as a treatment modality, the pediatrician needs to understand what the theory and treatment services are about.

Miller and colleagues believe that understanding the underlying sensory-motor systems involved in motor coordination and motor coordination disorders is necessary to develop an intervention plan. In the United States, the professionals trained to diagnose and treat SPDs are occupational therapists. The concept of an SPD refers to the inability to use information received through the senses in order to perform tasks needed in daily life. It is an umbrella term for 3 areas of possible difficulty: (1) the ability to process sensory inputs, which might be more intense or less intense than normal (if less intense, the body might seek to receive more stimulation or information); (2) the inability to or difficulty with discriminating different sensory inputs; and (3) the inability to perform the necessary motor behaviors.

The first step is sensory input and modulation of this input, then the brain must discriminate between different sensory inputs and, finally, the brain must perform the necessary motor behaviors. In performing these tasks, the brain might overrespond to the stimuli, underrespond to the stimuli, or seek more of the stimuli. These concepts lead to viewing an SPD as 1 of 3 types with subtypes of each (Box 5-1). Children with SPD react in similar ways to other sensory inputs, such as sights, sounds, smells, and tastes. As with the examples above, they overreact to such stimuli, ignore or underrespond to stimuli, or seek out stimuli.

## Box 5-1. Sensory Processing Disorders

### Sensory Modulation Disorder

Sensory modulation involves 3 primary sensory inputs: tactile, vestibular, and proprioception. Visual perception is not considered to be a primary part of the concept of sensory processing disorder; however, it is important. Children might overrespond to the stimuli, underrespond, or respond by seeking increased stimulation.

*Tactile (touch)*

- *Overrespond:* tactile defensiveness, avoids touching or being touched; dislikes certain textures of clothing or food
- *Underrespond:* may not know he has been touched; unaware of messy face, hands, clothes; misinterprets touch or texture
- *Sensory-seeking:* touches or hugs others; chews on shirt cuffs, rubs against objects, bumps into people

*Vestibular*

- *Overrespond:* avoids moving or being unexpectedly moved; insecure and anxious about falling or being off balance; car sickness
- *Underrespond:* does not notice or object to being moved; unaware of falling and protects self poorly
- *Sensory-seeking:* seeks fast and spinning movement and may not get dizzy; moves constantly and enjoys being upside down

*Proprioception*

- *Overrespond:* may be tight and uncoordinated; avoids activities that bring strong sensory input to muscles
- *Underrespond:* lacks inner drive to move for play; enjoys lifting, pushing, pulling, carrying heavy loads
- *Sensory-seeking:* craves bear hugs and being squeezed or pressed; seeks vigorous playground activities

### Sensory Discrimination Problems

These children may have difficulty distinguishing one sensation from another or in understanding what a sensation means. They might have difficulty recognizing that they have been touched or moved or become confused when turning or changing directions. They also might seem to be disconnected from their bodies, appearing to be clumsy or to bump into others. Similar problems might involve smell, taste, and temperature: They might not recognize familiar tastes or smells or not realize that it is cold or hot.

> **Box 5-1. Sensory Processing Disorders, continued**
>
> *Sensory-Based Motor Problems*
> These children might have difficulty with posture and balance, or they might have difficulty performing motor behaviors (dyspraxia). These behaviors might involve fine motor or gross motor skills. They might have difficulty learning a new, complex motor action, or they might have problems with coloring, cutting, writing, buttoning, zipping, or tying. They might also have problems in coordinating eating utensils, preferring to eat with their fingers.

# The Motor Coordination Disorder Medical Review of Systems

A reproducible worksheet with the following questions can be found in Appendix B.

The following medical review of systems incorporates the questions that might be asked under motor coordination disorder with those that might cover the broader aspects of an SPD.

## Relating to the concepts of SPD

**For the parents (or reworded for the child)**

*Visual Perception* questions
(Depending on age) "Does your child have problems when he must do quick eye-hand coordination tasks such as catch, hit, or throw a ball? Can he do puzzles?

Does your child knock things over or bump into things?"

*Proprioception* (fine motor/gross motor) questions
(Depending on age) "Does your child have difficulty with coloring or cutting? How about buttoning, zipping, or tying? Can your child manage the fork, knife, and spoon when eating or does your child prefer to eat with fingers?"

"Can your child run, jump, skip, climb as well as his or her friends?"

"How is your child's handwriting? Is it neat enough? Fast enough?"

"When playing sports, is your child coordinated? Does your child have difficulty with catching, hitting, throwing?"

*Tactile* questions

"Is your child sensitive to clothing. Does he or she complain about tags, elastic, socks, texture of clothes?"

"Does your child like to be held? Cuddled? What was it like when your child was an infant? What comforted your child then?"

*Vestibular* questions

(If age appropriate) "Can your child ride a two-wheel bike?"

"Can your child go up and down steps in tandem?"

"Does your child like to rest his or her head on an arm or to lean on the furniture arm or lie down?" (suggests weak upper trunk muscles)

# Treatment for Motor Coordination Disorder and Sensory Disorder

## Clinical Interventions

Treatment interventions focus on improving the identified area of motor difficulties. These interventions might be done by a physical therapist or an occupational therapist. All presenting problems should be treated. However, most occupational therapists who work within the school system will only address the handwriting problems.

Ideally, interventions will be part of the educational plan and will be provided within the school. If the school interventions focus only on the grapho-motor problems that result in difficulty with handwriting, parents may need to supplement these services with private occupational therapy services.

The interventions provided by an occupational therapist trained to apply the concepts of SPD will go beyond motor skills training. Since a pediatrician's patient might be receiving such services and most pediatricians are not familiar with such treatments, these treatment approaches will be discussed in more detail.

Occupational therapists trained to do so will develop intervention strategies to help children with SPD. The focus of therapy might be to improve a needed skill area, help minimize the overreaction to stimuli, or develop increased sensory input for underreactive stimuli.

The occupational therapist is critical to training parents how best to help their child. They are taught to adapt the child's environment to promote optimum functioning and to reduce disruption. Examples might be adaptations to daily routines (eg, dressing, bathing, transitions) to reduce the distress and discomfort associated with over- or underreacting or to assist the child in performing tasks known to be difficult. In addition, parents are taught ways to reduce some sources of sensation in the environment (eg, sounds, smells) or to develop consistent routines and predictability.

## Parent Education

The pediatrician, possibly along with the occupational therapist, will need to help explain to parents that these motor problems are neurologically based and that professional help is needed. As with learning disabilities and language disabilities, it is essential that parents understand how these problems affect the child and the family. They must learn how to compensate for their child's disabilities and to find ways to accommodate using their child's strengths. The pediatrician and occupational therapist may also need to help the parent explain these problems to the child's teacher and school.

Children with this disorder are confusing and difficult to understand. Why do they cry and resist when you wash their hair or brush their teeth? Why do they not like to be held or cuddled? Yet they might come up at times and give a hug. Why do they get angry if another child bumps into them? Yet they might go up and try to hug the same child? Why can't they learn to ride a bike like the other kids? Why do they avoid sports?

For example, children with SPD might have difficulty with sports activities involving running or such quick eye-hand coordination skills as catching, hitting, or throwing a ball. This child might not have the stamina or balance to do required skills. It is important to seek out peer interactions, activities, or sports that maximize the child's abilities and then compensate for the areas of disability.

Depending on the areas of disability, parents need to learn how to react and to handle their child. If the child is sensitive to touch, parents and others can learn how to touch or hold in a way that is more comfortable for the child. For example, alert the child to what they plan to do so that she can prepare. "Alice, I want to give you a hug. Are you ready?" Parents can be taught that the deep touch sensors are often less sensitive. Light strokes on the skin might be unpleasant, but deep hugs, pushing down on the muscles, might be fine.

Children who are tactile-defensive might feel the lack of touch and seek increased tactile stimulation, as long as they can prepare for it, initiate it, and control it. They might walk around touching or hugging other children. An occupational therapist might teach a parent how to stimulate the skin in an acceptable manner, satisfying the sense of tactile deprivation. Soft cloths or brushes might be rubbed over the arms or back. If done properly, the child relaxes and is more available to interact with the environment around him (school, home, etc).

Children with vestibular problems might have difficulty learning to ride a bike or to go down stairs in tandem. The upper back muscles are essential for maintaining an upright position against gravity. Often, because of inadequate signals from the brain, these children have weak upper trunk muscles. They like to rest their head on something or lie down rather than sit up. The child might become anxious if she feels off balance or feels a sudden change in body position. Escalators and elevators might create anxiety. Large, open spaces or hallways are difficult to handle because there are no close visual clues to use to judge where the body is.

It is not uncommon for children with vestibular perception difficulties to seek vestibular stimulation. They enjoy using the swing for extended times. They might like to spin in a chair or standing. Everyone else would be dizzy, but this child seems to enjoy the motion because it promotes relaxation.

## *Conclusion*

In this chapter the focus has been on motor coordination disorder. Because the authors believe that the pediatrician needs to understand the concepts of SPD, this model is also discussed.

When the clinical assessment and systems review questions support the impression of a motor coordination disorder, a referral to an occupational therapist may be made to assist in a more definitive diagnostic assessment and to help with treatment. If this occupational therapist is trained in the area of SPD, the evaluation will elaborate on these areas of concern and the recommended treatment plan will include interventions for these additional clinical problems.

# *Bibliography*

American Psychiatric Association. *Diagnostic and Statistical Manual of Mental Disorders.* 4th ed. Text rev. Washington, DC: American Psychiatric Association; 1994

Ayres AJ. *Sensory Integration and the Child.* Los Angeles, CA: Western Psychological Services; 1979

Bundy AC, Lane SJ, Murray EA, eds. *Sensory Integration Theory and Practice.* 2nd ed. Philadelphia, PA: F. A. Davis Company; 2002

Kranowitz CS. *The Out-Of-Sync-Child. Understanding and Coping with Your Sensory Processing Disorder.* New York, NY: Skylight Press; 2005

Michaud LJ; American Academy of Pediatrics Committee on Children With Disabilities. Prescribing therapy services for children with motor disabilities. *Pediatrics.* 2004;113:1836–1838

Myers SM, Johnson CP; American Academy of Pediatrics Council on Children With Disabilities. Management of children with autism spectrum disorders. *Pediatrics.* 2007;120:1162–118

# Chapter 6

# Confirming a Learning Disability and the Related Language or Motor Disability

The pediatrician plays a significant role as an advocate for children and their families. This role is essential for the child struggling in school. The pediatrician must advocate for the child and help to empower the parents to advocate as well.

For example, your office screening assessment supports the clinical impression of a possible learning disability. In addition, this assessment might suggest a language disability or a motor coordination disorder (sensory processing disorder). As with other clinical diagnostic impressions, the next step is to request the necessary follow-up studies needed to confirm your working clinical impressions.

To confirm the presence of a learning disability, a formal psychological and educational evaluation is needed. This battery of studies is referred to as a *psychoeducational evaluation.* A neuropsychological study might be done instead. A comprehensive speech-language evaluation, often including an audiological study, will clarify if there is a language disability; a comprehensive occupational therapy assessment will clarify if there is a motor coordination disorder (sensory processing disorder).

The data from these studies will also clarify the types of treatment interventions needed to address the existing disabilities. A medical treatment plan can then be established.

The assessment for problems in school follows the same medical assessment model as would be used for any other presenting problem.

1) Clinical data collection (chief complaint, history of present illness, history)
2) Review of systems

3)  Clinical and/or laboratory evaluations (eg, psychoeducational testing)
4)  Finalizing a clinical diagnosis
5)  Establishing a medical treatment plan

## *Obtaining the Necessary Evaluation Studies*

Under federal law, public schools are required to provide psychological and educational assessments of children when there is concern that there might be a learning disability. These laws will be reviewed in detail in Chapter 10. The procedure for the child's family requesting such assessments will be discussed later in this chapter. This process can be greatly facilitated if the child's pediatrician writes a brief note clarifying why such studies are needed. The studies are done by school professionals at no charge to the family.

Based on a 2004 revision to the federal Individuals with Disabilities Education Act (IDEA), a different assessment approach might be used by some school systems. This approach to assessment is called a *response to intervention (RTI)* model and will also be discussed later in this chapter.

Assessments can also be done by private practice providers. The quality of the test results should be the same whether done by public school professionals or private practice professionals. Should the family decide to use private professionals, a referral note from the pediatrician is very helpful. Often a letter from the pediatrician will maximize the possibility that the family's private health insurance plan will cover some or all of these assessment costs. Sample letters to request this are at the end of this chapter.

## *Initiating an Evaluation for a Learning Disability*

There are specific steps a parent must take to initiate a public school assessment for a possible learning disability. These steps are similar for assessment of suspected language and motor disabilities too, but they will be discussed separately within this chapter. Parents who have a child in a private school are also entitled to use the public school professionals for evaluation. In this case, they would initiate their request through the principal of the local public school where their child would have gone if not in a private school.

The first step is to present a letter to the principal of the school requesting an evaluation. As noted, a separate brief note from the child's pediatrician is helpful in reflecting the importance of the parent's request. Parents need to know that if a principal receives such a request in writing, the principal legally must respond back to the parents and must initiate a meeting to discuss the request within 10 calendar days. Although verbal requests should be taken seriously, they do not require such quick action. The note can be brief; for example

Dear ...:

My son, William, is in Ms Albert's third-grade class. He is struggling to keep up with the class work. I request that you set up a meeting to discuss the need for an assessment to clarify whether he has a learning disability.

(Signed)

If more details are available, they should be included in this letter. Encourage parents to be specific about these concerns. "My daughter received extra help with reading in second and third grades. She is now in fourth grade and is still struggling to comprehend what she reads." or "My son has difficulty with writing and shows problems with spelling and with punctuation." When possible, parents should cite something the teacher said in a parent conference that supports the concerns.

On receipt of the parent's letter, the principal or the professional responsible for special education services must set up a meeting. Parents, the child's classroom teacher(s), and appropriate school professionals should attend (school psychologist, learning disability specialist, school counselor, speech-language therapist, occupational therapist). At this meeting, the parents present their concerns. Any letters or other supporting documents are reviewed. It cannot be emphasized enough that a letter from the pediatrician is greatly valued at these meetings. This letter should summarize the results of the office evaluation, including the physical examination, relevant medical history, and the reasons for suspecting a possible disability. Any private evaluations should also be provided to the school professionals for review. At the end of this initial meeting, the school team will make recommendations. The decision might be to observe and work with the child longer before deciding to do a formal assessment or to proceed with the assessment. Should a full assessment be proposed, the specific tests to be done are identified, and parents are asked to give permission for these studies.

The IDEA 2004 law states that testing must be completed within 60 days of receiving parental consent for evaluation. Most states interpret this as 60 calendar days, but some will say it is 60 school days, or 60 calendar days minus the summers. A pediatrician should determine which approach is taken in his or her state. No matter what timeline is used, once the test data are complete, the principal calls another meeting with the parents and school professionals, where results of the evaluation are presented. Should the data support the diagnosis of a learning disability, these professionals will review what services and accommodations will be used to address the disabilities. No decisions can be finalized unless the parents agree. If they do, the school presents a contract, showing what will be done and how progress will be assessed. This contract is called an individualized education program (IEP). If parents do not agree with the proposed plan, they can appeal to the next level of decision-making. (Each of these steps will be discussed in more detail in Chapter 10.)

As mentioned, the latest revision of IDEA 2004, the federal law that governs special education, offers school systems another approach for assessing for a possible learning problem other than the comprehensive psychoeducational evaluation: the RTI evaluation. A summary of a psychoeducational evaluation and a response to intervention evaluation follows.

## The Psychoeducational Evaluation

Psychoeducational studies consist of a battery of tests that provide information on the child's overall abilities, particularly learning style, information processing, and academic skills. A significant part of this assessment is the IQ test, which helps clarify the student's strengths and weaknesses. It provides information regarding the student's ability to process verbally and visually presented information as well as his or her overall intellectual potential. Considerable additional information is derived from the IQ test relating to sequencing abilities, short- and long-term memory issues, language functioning, and processing speed. The most widely recognized IQ test is the Wechsler Intelligence Scale for Children (WISC). The corresponding version for preschoolers is the Wechsler Preschool and Primary Scale of Intelligence

(WPPSI). For students older than 16 years, there is the Wechsler Adult Intelligence Scale (WAIS). In addition to the IQ test, the examiner might perform specific tests to evaluate the student's cognitive abilities, especially tests of memory and organizational skills.

The other parts of the psychoeducational evaluation assess the student's academic skills: reading, written language, and math. There are many standardized tests that can be used to obtain this information. These studies include brief tasks and, for older students, more complex activities consistent with grade demands (eg, reading multiple paragraphs, writing essays). Studies might include informal measures but should also involve standardized tests that provide objective scores that can be compared with grade-level expectations, as well as to the student's intellectual potential. Testing should also allow comparison of the student's performance under timed and untimed conditions. The most frequently used battery of educational testing is the Woodcock-Johnson Psychoeducational Battery.

## Neuropsychological Evaluation

Schools will provide psychoeducational testing. Neuropsychological evaluations are done in the private sector. Psychoeducational testing in the school system is done by a school psychologist and/or a special educator. The evaluation is aimed at identifying a child's qualifying condition for services or supportive services in the school system. These evaluations highlight a child's strengths and weaknesses, defer to the student support team to determine eligibility, and contain limited recommendations.

A neuropsychological evaluation usually contains some of the same measures done during psychoeducational testing (such as IQ testing). However, it goes into more detailed assessment of executive function, memory, visual-spatial processing, visual-motor processing, language function, effort, attention and, in some cases, personality function. The evaluation goes beyond the "numbers" to assess a child's approach to the task. The results are interpreted within the context of having an appreciation for brain behavior relationships and how central nervous system dysfunction may present functional deficits. From these results, more specific recommendations can be made for the child in and out of the school setting. Schools are not required to accept the results and recommendations of any "independent evaluation."

Most schools, however, are usually receptive to the findings, though they might not follow all of the recommendations.

Neuropsychological evaluations are not always covered by medical insurance and can be very expensive. In general, insurance companies will cover this testing when a child has an underlying disorder that puts him at risk of a learning disability. This might include chromosomal disorder; hydrocephalus; sickle cell anemia (high risk for strokes); or a history of prematurity, lead poisoning, head injury, or cranial irradiation. Neuropsychological evaluation might also be recommended in the case of a child who is struggling in school after being identified as needing support and receiving services. As always, a letter of recommendation from the pediatrician supporting this testing is usually necessary (sample letters are at the end of this chapter).

## The Response to Intervention Assessment

This approach to assessing a student who is struggling in school is a 3-step process. Each step involves a more detailed intervention.

1) If a student is struggling academically, the classroom teacher is asked to try additional teaching approaches to help the student master the expected material.

2) If the student still does not make progress, a second level of intervention is tried. Here, a support teacher with special training in addressing learning problems assists the classroom teacher and works individually with the student.

3) Should the student still not make progress, IDEA 2004 states that an IEP is written and the student is assigned to receive special education services.

The rules and regulations established by the US Department of Education for implementing this RTI approach encourages school systems to do a comprehensive psychoeducational evaluation or equivalent studies to clarify the reasons for the difficulties before deciding what programs or services are needed. Intervention steps 1 and 2 do not clarify if the school problems are the result of specific learning disabilities; the child's level of intellectual functioning; or the impact of bilingual issues, environmental or family stresses, or a possible specific psychiatric disorder such as pervasive developmental disorder.

For these reasons, most school professionals believe that it is not possible to write an IEP or to decide the best placement for a child who is struggling in school without first clarifying the reasons for the problems. Thus, as noted previously, between steps 2 and 3, formal studies should be done.

## Evaluation for a Language Disability

If parents use their public school system, they would use the same steps requesting an evaluation that have been described. The committee in this case would recommend a speech and language evaluation. Some parents might prefer to see a private speech-language therapist for these studies, then provide the reports to the school system.

Whether done by the school system or privately, these assessments will explore for difficulties in all areas of speech and language. The studies should clarify if there is an articulation problem resulting in errors in sound production, use, representation, or organization. Examples of this would be substitutions of one sound for another or omission of sounds. Still other studies should clarify if there might be an oral-motor problem resulting in poor speech or if the child might have a problem with stuttering. Further studies explore for a possible receptive and/or expressive language disability.

If any of these speech or language disabilities are found, specific treatment plans are described as well as any accommodations needed in the classroom. These services should be offered by the school system. Parents might elect to use private professionals instead of or in addition to the services provided by the school system.

Most receptive and expressive language disabilities are the result of phonological processing difficulties. These same phonological processing abilities are needed to learn basic reading and writing skills. Thus, if phonological processing problems are noted by the speech-language therapist and formal educational studies have not yet been done, the pediatrician should recommend such studies.

## Evaluation for a Motor Disability

If it is suspected that the child or adolescent has a fine motor or gross motor problem that is impacting on learning, an occupational therapist and possibly a physical therapist can assess to confirm such a clinical impression and to establish a treatment intervention. If the therapist is part of the school system, interventions might focus only on handwriting. An occupational therapist in private practice will work on this fine motor problem as well as on related problems (coloring, cutting, buttoning, zipping, tying, controlling eating utensils). The private practice occupational therapist might also work on gross motor problems that interfere with skills needed for sports or other activities. If this occupational therapist has been trained in the concepts of sensory processing disorder, a broader plan of help may be developed.

## The Pediatrician's Role in the Assessment Process

The pediatrician might be the first person to suspect that the child's struggles and behaviors in school might be secondary to an unrecognized and untreated area of disability. Or, the child's family may have had studies done in the past and already know of these disabilities. The pediatrician, as the child's advocate, can facilitate getting the necessary studies done and the appropriate treatment interventions started.

If the office screening is the first clue suggestive of a possible disability, the child's parents should be advised of the studies needed and the services that their public school system should provide. A letter summarizing your findings and explaining why further studies or services are needed will provide support for the parents as they move through the public school system.

Should the parents want to have these studies done privately, they will quickly learn that many health insurance plans unfortunately will not cover the cost for evaluations or therapy related to learning disabilities. The general philosophy is that school problems are not medical problems. Some health insurance plans may resist covering speech and language or occupational therapy evaluations as well. If the pediatrician writes a letter in support of such studies, some insurance plans may agree to cover some or all of the cost for the assessment.

The pediatrician's letter needs to stress that such studies are "medically necessary to finalize the medical diagnosis and to assist in designing the necessary medical treatment plan." The stress needs to be that the child has a neurologically based disorder. If there is relevant medical history supporting the possibility of neurologic impairment, it should be listed. Examples would be lead poisoning, head injury, etc. Sample letters for each situation follow.

## Box 6-1. Sample Assessment Request Letter

I have been following William in my practice. Based on my informal assessment, I find clinical evidence that he might have a learning disability. Thus I request that the professionals at his school do the necessary studies to clarify if my clinical impressions are correct.

## Box 6-2. Sample Letters

*Psychoeducational or Neuropsychological*

"Cathy Anderson is a patient in my practice. Based on my clinical assessment, she shows evidence of *neurologically based* processing deficits. It is *medically essential* that psychoeducational testing be done to clarify these areas of disability. Only with such data will I be able to prepare a comprehensive *medical treatment plan*. I request that the insurance plan cover the cost for these essential studies."

*Speech-Language*

"John Williams is a patient in my practice. Based on my clinical assessment, he shows evidence of a *neurologically based* language disability manifested by both receptive and expressive language deficits. A comprehensive speech and language evaluation is necessary to clarify these areas of disability. Only with such data will I be able to finalize a *medical diagnosis* and to develop a *medical treatment plan*."

*Occupational Therapy*

"Alice Cohen is a patient in my practice. Based on my clinical assessment, she has a *neurologically based* motor coordination disorder manifested by fine motor, gross motor, and visual-motor difficulties as well as clinical evidence suggestive of a vestibular disorder. A comprehensive occupational therapy evaluation is necessary for me to clarify these areas of disability, finalize a *medical diagnosis,* and prepare a *medical treatment plan*."

## Conclusion

The office screening assessment will alert the pediatrician to a possible learning disability, language disability, or motor coordination disorder (sensory processing disorder). At this time, the physician needs to refer the family to the appropriate programs or professionals to clarify if the diagnosis is correct and, if so, to recommend the necessary treatment plans.

The pediatrician, as the child's and the family's advocate, plays a critical role in clarifying these possible diagnoses and in facilitating the necessary assessments. Only with such data can an appropriate medical and educational intervention plan be developed. The pediatrician also must help to empower parents to advocate for their child within the school system and with their medical insurance plan.

## Bibliography

American Psychiatric Association. *Diagnostic and Statistical Manual of Mental Disorders.* 4th ed. Text rev. Washington, DC: American Psychiatric Association; 1994

Latham PS, Latham H, Mandlewitz M. *Special Education Law.* Washington, DC: JKL Communications; 2008

Silver LB. *The Misunderstood Child. Understanding and Coping with Your Child's Learning Disabilities.* 4th ed. New York, NY: Three Rivers Press; 2006

US Department of Education. *Building the Legacy: IDEA 2004.* US Department of Education Web site. http://idea.ed.gov/explore/home

Wright PWD, Wright PD. *Special Education Law.* 2nd ed. Hartfield, VA: Harbor House Law Press; 2008

# Part II

# Related Disorders

# Chapter 7

# ▶ The Impact of Learning Beyond the School: Secondary Emotional, Social, and Family Problems

Learning disabilities may interfere with mastery of academic skills or class participation. Grades might drop. Teachers become concerned. Parents may become upset. It is clear that learning disabilities are school disabilities. It is equally important to understand that *learning disabilities are also life disabilities.* The same learning problems that interfere with reading, writing, or math may interfere with baseball, basketball, riding a bike, doing chores at home, or making conversation with peers.

This child might have difficulties making friends or participating in peer activities. If parents do not understand that learning disabilities are life disabilities, they become upset with behaviors at home or the child's apparent refusal to do specific tasks. If the child cannot make small talk, participate in expected activities, or act as expected, siblings might become angry for the same reasons that the kids at school get angry.

For these reasons, learning disabilities result in secondary emotional, social, and family problems. These problems are secondary because they are a reflection of the frustrations and failures the child experiences in life. In addition, children with learning disabilities are at high risk of having other associated neurologic conditions that might impact on the lives of those around them (eg, attention-deficit/hyperactivity disorder). These associated disorders will be discussed in Chapter 8.

The special education professional will know the child's areas of learning ability and disability in order to develop the necessary educational programs. Parents often are not taught their child's areas of strength and weakness. Without this information, they will have difficulty knowing what sports or activities their child is most likely to succeed in, what chores to assign, what camps to select, and what decisions to make in countless other crucial daily situations. Knowledge of a child's strengths and weaknesses helps parents maximize activities and experiences where the child might succeed and minimize activities and experiences that might lead to frustration and failure. It is important for pediatricians to appreciate this reality: learning disabilities are life disabilities.

# Information Processing

A model based on how the brain processes information is helpful in illustrating the impact learning disabilities have on life activities. In a basic form, this model describes how information is received, processed, and used.

- Input: Receiving information through auditory or visual pathways
- Integration: Once received, the ability to sequence, understand, organize, and use information
- Memory: Storage of information as well as retrieval of information received by auditory or visual pathways
- Output: Getting information out through motor activity or through oral language

  Each of these is illustrated in further detail as follows.

## Input Disabilities

A child or adolescent with visual perception difficulties may have problems with sports activities that require quick eye-hand coordination, such as catching, throwing, or hitting a ball. This ball could be a baseball, basketball, or any other sports ball. The first task requires eye-hand coordination. The child must look in the right direction and spot the ball—a visual-figure-ground skill. The child with a disability in this area may not spot the ball and stand there as the ball hits the ground. The second task is to keep one's eye on the ball. Doing this enables the brain to use depth perception to track the ball and to inform the body, legs, arms, and hands where to be at the right time to catch the ball. Children with visual perception problems might play these sports poorly and, thus, avoid them. They might intuitively learn that they do best in sports that do not require such eye-hand, eye-foot coordination (eg, swimming, soccer, certain track and field events, horseback riding).

What about jump rope? First the child must spot where the rope hits the ground (visual figure-ground). Then, the child must focus on this spot while running toward the rope so that depth perception can be used to tell the body when and where to jump. This child might have similar problems with four-square, hopscotch, and other activities.

A child with depth perception problems may fall off their seat, bump into things, or misjudge the distance to a drink and knock over the glass. He or she may be confused by large, open spaces such as gyms, parking lots, or shopping malls.

A child with an auditory perception problem might misunderstand what adults or friends say and thus respond incorrectly. This child might have difficulty knowing what sounds to listen to when there are competing sounds; thus, miss what is being said by parents or friends. If the child has a delay in processing language, he or she might become confused and appear to tune out.

## Integration Disabilities

Children with sequencing problems might confuse the steps involved in playing a game, might hit a baseball and run to the wrong base, or have difficulty getting into uniform. Imagine a basketball coach's response when he explains a practice drill and the child messes up because he cannot remember the sequence of tasks involved.

Much of humor is based on processing the subtle meaning of words or phrases. A child with abstraction difficulties might miss the meaning of jokes or idioms.

A child has difficulty organizing information, procedures, or materials. These organizational problems may create family conflicts. The child's bedroom is disorganized and things are left around the house. He or she might not bring the right material home to do homework or might forget to return these items to school to be turned in.

## Memory Disabilities

Children with short-term memory disabilities might have difficulty communicating in a social interaction. They might meet someone they know but forget the name. A parent gives this child a series of tasks and becomes upset when only the first one is done. A friend tells this child to meet after school and to walk home together and the child forgets.

A child studies for a test, really knowing the material. The next day, the information is not retained and he or she does poorly on a test. The teacher believes the child did not study.

## Output Disabilities

The inability to write quickly and legibly or to spell can be a problem with certain games, performing some activities, taking telephone messages, or writing a note to a friend. Fine motor difficulties can cause problems with buttoning, tying, zipping, playing certain games, or cutting food. This child looks and acts differently when doing many life tasks.

Expressive language problems make communication with family and friends difficult. A child with an output disability might have problems with small talk or with interacting in a conversation. He or she might appear to be shy, avoiding talking or being with people for fear of saying the wrong thing and appearing foolish.

## *Secondary Emotional Problems*

As can be seen, learning disabilities impact all aspects of life. The frustrations and failures in school, with peers, and within the family might lead to secondary emotional problems. These emotional problems will present clinically in different ways. Some children will internalize these stresses, some will externalize these stresses, and some may somatize these stresses.

### Internalize Stress

These children are aware of their difficulties and experience anxiety, depression, and/or increased anger. They might present with an anxiety disorder, clinical depression, or problems with anger control. These disorders are discussed in Chapter 13.

### Externalize Stress

Some children find the discomfort and pain of stress with the resulting anxiety and depression too much to cope with. They decide not to cope with this stress by "getting rid of it." They externalize the anxiety and depression. To do this, they project their problems onto others, accepting little or no responsibility for the problems. Suddenly their behavior or academic difficulties are because of others. "The teacher ignored me when I asked for help." A child did this or caused that. Their brother set them up. They might get into a fight but try to explain why it was started by someone else.

By projecting all of the blame onto others, the child does not have to accept responsibility for his problems. He often feels little or no anxiety or depression. However, all of the meaningful adults in his life—parents, teachers—feel anxious and worried about him. Since this child accepts no responsibility for problems, it is difficult to get him to agree that help is needed.

According to the *Diagnostic and Statistical Manual of Mental Disorders, Fourth Edition, Text Revision,* children who externalize their problems are seen as having 1 of 2 types of disorders. If they externalize their problems primarily within the family but possibly in the school—challenging rules, getting into difficulties and then blaming others, being oppositional and defiant—they are said to have an *oppositional defiant disorder* (Box 7-1). If the stresses are not relieved, these behaviors might expand beyond the family, leading to challenging school and society rules, fighting, stealing, and possibly breaking the law. This child is said to have a *conduct disorder* (Box 7-2).

---

**Box 7-1. Diagnostic Criteria for Oppositional Defiant Disorder**

A. The child shows a pattern of negativistic, hostile, and defiant behavior lasting at least six months, during which for or more of the following are present:
   (1) Often loses temper
   (2) Often argues with adults
   (3) Often actively defies or refuses to comply with adults' requests or rules
   (4) Often deliberately annoys people
   (5) Often blames others for his or her mistakes or misbehaviors
   (6) Is often touchy or easily annoyed by others
   (7) Is often angry and resentful
   (8) Is often spiteful or vindictive

B. The disturbance in behavior causes clinically significant impairment in social, academic, or occupational functioning.

C. The behaviors do not occur exclusively during the course of a Psychotic or Mood Disorder.

D. Criteria are not met for Conduct Disorder and, if the indivual is age 18 years or older, criteria are not met for Antisocial Personality Disorder.

---

Reprinted from: Americam Psychiatric Association: *Diagnostic and Statistical Manual of Mental Disorders,* Fourth Edition, Text Revision. Washington DC: American Psychiatric Association; 2000:102.

## Box 7-2. Diagnostic Criteria for Conduct Disorder

A. A repetitive and persistent pattern of behavior in which the basic rights of others or major age-appropriate societal norms or rules are violated, as manifested by the presence of 3 (or more) of the following criteria in the past 12 months, with at least one criterion present in the past 6 months

*Aggression to people and animals.*
　(1) Often bullies, threatens, or intimidates others
　(2) Often initiates physical fights
　(3) Has used a weapon that can cause serious physical harm to others (eg, a bat, brick, broken bottle, knife, gun)
　(4) Has been physically cruel to people
　(5) Has been physically cruel to animals
　(6) Has stolen while confronting a victim (eg, mugging, purse snatching, extortion, armed robbery)
　(7) Has forced someone into sexual activity

*Destruction of property*
　(8) Has deliberately engaged in fire setting with the intent of causing serious damage
　(9) Has deliberately destroyed others' property (other than fire setting)

*Deceitfulness or theft*
　(10) Has broken into someone else's house, building, or car
　(11) Often lies to obtain goods or favors or to avoid obligations (ie, "cons" others)
　(12) Has stolen items of nontrivial value without confronting a victim (eg, shoplifting, but without breaking and entering; forgery)

*Serious violations of rules*
　(13) Often stays out at night despite parental prohibitions, beginning before age thirteen
　(14) Has run away from home overnight at least twice while living in a parental or parental-surrogate home (or once without returning for a lengthy period)
　(15) Often truant from school (beginning before age thirteen)
B. The disturbance in behavior causes clinically significant impairment in social, academic, or occupational functioning.
C. If the individual is 18 years or older, criteria are not met for Antisocial Personality Disorder.

Reprinted from: Americam Psychiatric Association: *Diagnostic and Statistical Manual of Mental Disorders,* Fourth Edition, Text Revision. Washington DC: American Psychiatric Association; 2000:98–99.

It is important to understand that these disorders are a reflection of underlying stress and how the child copes with this stress. Interventions must focus on the causes of the stress as well as on the negative behaviors.

## Somatize Stress

Often these physical symptoms are vague and difficult to understand or to assess. They might have a general eating problem, being a picky eater, over-eating, or eating too little. Some may develop specific eating disorders such as bulimia or anorexia. They might have somatic complaints, complaining of a headache or a stomachache. Others might develop other physical symptoms, often involving the gastrointestinal system.

## *Secondary Social Problems*

Social problems might be secondary to the frustrations and failures resulting from the learning, language, or motor disabilities. These will be discussed in this chapter. Other social skills problems seem to be another result of a dysfunctional nervous system (ie, they are also neurologically based). These pragmatic social skills problems will be discussed in Chapter 9.

As described, learning disabilities are life disabilities. These learning disabilities impact peer interactions, activities, sports, and life in general. Many children and adolescents with learning disabilities have problems interacting socially. These social skills problems are secondary to their disabilities.

How these social problems are reflected depends on age and gender. As an example, let's think of a 10-year-old child who has difficulties with visual perception, visual motor skills, and gross motor coordination but has excellent listening and talking skills. If this 10-year-old is a boy, he will be in trouble socially. Boys interact and bond through activities, usually through sports. Most do not usually relate or interact by talking. This child goes out with his classmates or neighbors but cannot play the usual organized sports, such as baseball or basketball, well enough to keep up. He may be teased or not selected to play. Soon he finds it easier to stay at home and to avoid peer interactions. At school he might walk around the edges of the playground during recess. His social problems are a result of the impact of his learning disabilities on the skills required for sports. What else might he do? He might realize that younger children prefer to run, climb, and ride bikes. He can manage these skills. In addition, the younger children will look up to him while his peers avoid or tease him. He prefers to spend his playtime with younger children or to stay in the house.

Now suppose that this 10-year-old is a girl. She might quickly learn that she is not good at sports and avoid such activities. We want girls to participate in sports; however, girls relate in other ways as well. Ten-year-old girls usually bond by talking. It is common for several girls to sit and talk about everything. She has good language skills and does very well, so this girl may have fewer social problems.

## Secondary Family Problems

*When one member of a family hurts, everyone in the family feels the pain.* For this reason, when a child with learning disabilities is not recognized, diagnosed, and provided help, he or she becomes frustrated and hurts. Soon parents and siblings feel the impact of this pain and develop their own problems. Parents are upset about the lack of apparent effort or progress. If the disabilities have been identified and the parents have not been educated about the impact these disabilities have on life and not just on learning, they become upset. Without understanding, parents might become angry about behaviors the child may not be able to help. Sometimes, one parent becomes firm and strict and the other parent becomes soft and permissive. Parents might begin to clash. Siblings get angry about the stresses this child causes or because this sibling gets more attention. They might complain about double standards of responsibility.

Learning disabilities might interfere with listening and responding to parents' instructions or requests. Certain chores might be difficult to remember or to do. For example, the child with fine motor and visual motor difficulties might have difficulty with buttoning clothes or tying shoes. She is seen as lazy or as wanting a parent to take care of her. This child might have difficulty with peers and prefer to sit at home than to play with friends or to join a sports team. Parents become upset.

It is essential that the child's parents understand the learning disabilities as well as the teacher or the members of the special education team. Parents must understand the child's areas of learning disabilities and areas of learning ability. With this knowledge, they might be able to select the right chores to be done, to give instructions in a way that is understood, and to pick the right sport or activity for their child.

These concepts for helping parents will be discussed in more detail in Chapter 13.

## Conclusion

When assessing for a behavioral or emotional problem, it is essential that the pediatrician attempt to clarify if the presenting problems are primary or secondary. Did the behaviors begin at a certain time or do they occur only in certain situations? Or, have these behaviors been present at different times throughout the child's life and do these behaviors occur in all situations and at all times? The interventions may be different for each situation.

Most essential is that the pediatrician help the family understand that learning, language, and motor disabilities are life disabilities. Unless the total child is understood in his or her total environment, there will be less than successful progress. It is important to understand how the processing problems might be interfering with the child's ability to be successful at home, with peers, and in activities. If the child has social skills difficulties, it is necessary to determine if they are secondary to learning, language, or motor disabilities, or if they are yet another reflection of a dysfunctional nervous system, a pragmatic social skills disability.

## Bibliography

American Psychiatric Association. *Diagnostic and Statistical Manual of Mental Disorders.* 4th ed. Text rev. Washington, DC: American Psychiatric Association; 2000

Silver LB. *The Misunderstood Child. Understanding and Coping with Your Child's Learning Disabilities.* 4th ed. New York, NY: Three Rivers Press; 2006

# Chapter 8

# Related Neurologically Based Disorders

National survey studies show that there is a continuum of neurologically based disorders often associated with learning disabilities. Between 30% and 50% of children with learning disabilities will have one or more of the other disorders within this continuum.

As noted in Chapter 7, if the emotional problems are secondary to the learning disabilities, the behaviors start at a certain time and occur in certain situations. On the contrary, when the behaviors reflect a neurologically based disorder, there is a chronic and a pervasive history of the difficulties. Often there is a family history of similar patterns.

The basic neuro-architecture of the brain is in place and functioning early in pregnancy, possibly by the sixth week. This process of brain development is controlled and directed by the genetic code. The specific steps involved are carried out by messengers produced by and directed by the genes called *neuroendocrine proteins.* Each connects with a specific cell and instructs it what to do. Once the tasks are complete, each specific neuroendocrine stops functioning. Another is produced to carry out the next steps in neurodevelopment. It is thought that problems with brain structure might be the result of genetic problems or of what are referred to as *neuroendocrine disruptors*—something that interferes with neuroendocrine expression.

In most areas of the brain, no new neurons are formed after birth. However, the architecture of the brain is modified by pruning of areas in less use and increased axon and dendrite connections in areas of increased use. This process of pruning and rewiring is especially active during the first several years of life. In addition to the genetic influence on brain development, the brain is critically sensitive to both the positive and the negative influences of its environment.

It is suspected that the basis for this continuum of neurologically based disorders relates to the complexity of brain development and maturation. If something disrupts development in utero or during further brain development after birth, more than one area of the brain may be affected. Thus there may be multiple clinical outcomes.

## Continuum of Neurologically Based Disorders

Statistical studies show that if someone has any one of the following disorders, there is a 30% to 50% possibility that he or she will have one or more of the other disorders.

1) Other cortically based disorders
   - Learning disability
   - Language disability
   - Motor disability
2) Attention-deficit/hyperactivity disorder (ADHD)
3) Emotional regulatory disorders
   - Anxiety disorders
   - Depression
   - Anger-control disorder
   - Obsessive-compulsive disorder
4) Tic disorders
5) Bipolar disorder

Thus if any one of these disorders is identified, it is essential that each of the others be considered and ruled in or out. The statistical likelihood of finding one or more of these other disorders is too great not to do such an assessment.

General pediatricians frequently assess and diagnose a child with ADHD. When this is done, it is critical to assess whether any of the other disorders within the continuum are present. It is not uncommon for the ADHD to be identified and treated, yet the child continues to perform poorly in school. Later, a learning, language, or motor disability surfaces as well. Once these problems are addressed, the child improves.

If anxiety, depression, or anger-control problems are noted, it is essential that the pediatrician determine whether the problems observed are secondary to the initially diagnosed learning disabilities or if they are independent of this initially diagnosed disorder. The approach to interventions will be different for each.

# Clinical Review of the Related Disorders

## Cortically Based Disorders

Learning disabilities, language disabilities, and sensory processing disorders are discussed throughout this book.

## Attention-Deficit/Hyperactivity Disorder

Because of this comorbidity, if a child is diagnosed with ADHD it is important to assess for a possible cortical-based disorder. To treat ADHD and not address other disabilities will result in a less than successful intervention.

## Emotional Regulatory Disorders

It is not uncommon for children with learning disabilities to struggle with anxiety, depression, or anger control as a result of the frustrations and failures experienced and the impact these experiences have on self-esteem and self-image. If the emotional problems are secondary to the learning disabilities, the clinical history will show that they started at a certain time and occur in specific situations but not in all situations.

For 30% to 50% of children with learning disabilities, problems regulating emotions are not situational but are neurologically based. Thus the clinician will find a chronic and pervasive history and often a family history.

### Anxiety Disorders

Anxiety is an emotional uneasiness associated with irrational anticipation of something bad happening or of danger. It is distinguished from fear, the emotional response to real danger, although the somatic responses to both are the same.

Children may show a general feeling of anxiety. They may have excessive and unrealistic worries about competence, approval, appropriateness of past behavior, and the future. Others may show a specific type of anxiety. They may have separation anxiety, where they feel anticipatory uneasiness about separating from parents or other loved ones. Or they may develop a phobia, resulting in avoiding behaviors and functional and social impairment. Common phobias seen in children include fear of animals in general, cats, dogs, blood, fire, germs, dirt, height, insects, small or closed spaces, snakes, spiders, strangers, and thunder.

Other children develop a specific pattern of anxiety. They may show social anxiety and experience significant anxiety provoked by exposure to certain types of social or performance situations, often leading to avoidance behaviors. Following a traumatic experience, a child may develop post-traumatic stress disorder, making the child anxious and overly cautious. The child may reexperience the traumatic event accompanied by symptoms of increased arousal and avoidance of stimuli associated with the trauma.

The anxiety level in some children gets so high that a fight-or-flight response is triggered, causing a panic attack lasting up to 30 minutes or more. Panic attacks are accompanied by a sudden onset of intense apprehension, fearfulness, or terror, and are often associated with feelings of impending doom. During these attacks the body responds with symptoms such as shortness of breath, heart palpitations, chest pain or discomfort, choking or smothering sensations, and fear of "going crazy" or of losing control.

A summary of the most common behaviors a child might experience if he or she has an anxiety disorder include

1) Cardiac: palpitations, tachycardia, increase in blood pressure, flushing or pallor
2) Respiratory: feelings of shortness of breath, increased rate of breathing
3) Skin: blotching, rash, increase in skin temperature with sweating, funny sensations felt in the skin
4) Muscles: mild tremor, muscle tension, muscle cramps
5) Other: headache, chest pain, over-alertness, startling easily, insomnia, nightmares, dizziness, fainting, urinary frequency
6) Psychological behaviors: talk of fears, feeling scared, tense, nervous, upset, stressed, fretful, restless, can't think clearly
7) Social behaviors: appears clingy, needy, dependent, shy, withdrawn, uneasy

## Depression

*It is normal for children to experience depressed moods as they mature out of one stage of development and move to another.* Each major growth milestone experienced by a child is associated with some anxiety about the new tasks and sadness about giving up the comfort of the previous stage. The toddler learns to walk and can finally get around without help. There is the fear of moving out alone, and there is the sadness of leaving behind a special kind of closeness and dependency. During adolescence, there is a similar psychological process as the teen experiences the anxiety of growing up and accepting new responsibilities and the sadness of giving up the special experiences and safety of childhood. So, too, a child might experience grief after the loss of a parent, grandparent, or other relative. These examples are defined as adjustment disorders.

Some children experience feelings of depression that do not to relate to any situation or reason, and start and stop with no apparent explanations. Such behavior may prompt parents to seek further evaluation.

Symptoms associated with depression are

1) Depressed or irritable mood
2) Diminished interest or loss of pleasure in almost all activities
3) Sleep disturbance
4) Weight change or appetite disturbance
5) Decreased concentration or indecisiveness
6) Suicidal ideation or thoughts of death
7) Agitation or slowness of thinking
8) Fatigue or loss of energy
9) Feelings of worthlessness or inappropriate guilt
10) Irritability and increased anger

In the *Diagnostic and Statistical Manual of Mental Disorders, Fourth Edition, Text Revision* (DSM-IV-TR), 2 specific types of depressive disorders are described. If the child shows a depressed or irritable mood that lasts a year or longer and the individual is never truly symptom-free for more than 2 months, the depression is called *dysthymia*. Symptoms include changes in appetite and sleep, decreased energy, low self-esteem, difficulty making decisions or poor concentration, and/or feelings of hopelessness.

The second type of depression is called a *major depression,* which is manifested by difficulty regulating several moods. Although depressed, he or she may at times go into a euphoric and excited state (hypomania or mania), characterized by an abnormal and persistently elevated, expansive, or irritable mood. He or she might have an inflated self-esteem or feelings of grandiosity, decreased need for sleep, pressure of speech, flight of ideas, distractibility, increased involvement in goal-directed activities, or psychomotor agitation. This hypomanic state might last minutes, hours, or a week or more if not treated. If a person experiences mood swings with major periods of depression and hypomania, the term *bipolar disorder* is used. If the person only experiences mood swings from normality to depression, the term *unipolar disorder* is used. (Adults may experience each of these mood swings for days or weeks. Children usually experience these mood swings for minutes or hours, often showing frequent mood swings.)

### Anger Control

The clinical term for this disorder is *intermittent explosive disorder.* The angry outbursts go beyond the typical tantrum. Parents often refer to these episodes as "melt downs."

The child will quickly lose his or her temper, often so quickly that it is not clear what sets it off. This rage reaction may last for 5 to 10 minutes to up to an hour. During an episode, the child might be screaming, cursing, hitting, throwing, or threatening. The behavior seems to be irrational, and the child cannot be reasoned with or stopped. The episode ends almost as quickly as it begins. Once over, the child may feel sorry for what he or she did and have difficulty explaining their behavior. The child might explain, "I don't know why I did that. It felt like I was sitting in my head, watching myself."

Usually, children with intermittent explosive disorder only have melt downs at home or when out with a parent. They usually do not occur in school, with peers, or during activities. Thus it is easy to suspect that the anger must be related to family issues. It seems that the underlying problem is that the child has a less than normal ability to control anger. In school or with friends, there may be little to make the child angry and the child might not want to embarrass himself. In contrast, at home there might be many things that make the child angry ("turn off TV," "do your homework," or "hang up your coat"). The child may make little effort to control his anger. The level of anger rises and leads to the melt down.

## Obsessive-Compulsive Disorder

Obsessions are unwanted thoughts, images, or impulses that the individual realizes are senseless or unnecessary, intrude into his or her consciousness involuntarily, and cause functional impairment and distress. Despite this lack of control, the child still recognizes that these thoughts originate in his or her own mental process. Since they arise in the mind, obsessions can take the form of any mental event (eg, simple repetitive words, thoughts, fears, memories, pictures, or elaborate dramatic scenes).

Compulsions are actions that are responses to a perceived internal obligation to follow certain rituals or rules. They also cause functional impairment. Compulsions may be motivated directly by obsessions or efforts to ward off certain thoughts, impulses, or fears. Children may report compulsions without the perception of a mental component. Like obsessions, compulsions are often viewed as being unnecessary, excessive, or senseless, and involuntary or forced. Individuals suffering from compulsions will often elaborate a variety of precise rules for the chronology, rate, order, duration, and number of repetitions of their act.

A person with obsessive-compulsive disorder may have obsessions, compulsions, or both, resulting in difficulty functioning. She or he feels forced or invaded by the symptoms and perceives the senselessness or excessiveness of the thoughts or acts. Although the child might try to ignore or suppress the thoughts or actions, the anxiety builds and the behaviors break through.

Common behaviors in individuals who have obsessive-compulsive disorder include

1) Counting or repeating behavior: the need to touch something a certain number of times or an even or odd number of times; the need to repeat a specific behavior or pattern of behaviors; the need to count certain things until finished

2) Checking or questioning behavior: the need to check and recheck something (that the front door is locked, the stove is off, the car keys were brought in, the closet light is off); the need to ask a question a specific number of times or until the person answers in the exact way it is needed to be heard

3) Arranging and organizing behaviors: the need to tie shoes or to dress or undress in a certain sequence or certain way; the need to organize toys or dolls or other items in a certain way; becoming upset if anything is changed

4) Cleaning and/or washing behaviors: the need to lather and rinse an exact number of times while showering or to brush one's hair a certain number of times in a certain pattern; the need to wash one's hands repeatedly; the need to take frequent showers or to change clothes

5) Perfectionism: the need to correct what is done over and over, seeking for it to be perfect as the child sees it (Students might write something and then need to erase and redo it over and over, striving to make it look right or to cover the task perfectly.)

These obsessions and/or compulsions may begin to appear at age 6 or 7, sometimes earlier. They may decrease in intensity at times but return later. Often there is a family history.

## Tic Disorders

These disorders are familiar to pediatricians. Thus they will only be reviewed in general in this book. A tic is a sudden, repetitive movement, gesture, or utterance that typically mimics some aspect of normal behavior. Usually of brief duration, individual tics rarely last more than a second. They tend to occur in spurts and at times have a convulsion-like characteristic. Individual tics can occur singly or together in an orchestrated pattern. They can vary in their frequency and forcefulness. These tics seem to come and go over time and to change in form. Although many tics can be temporarily suppressed, they are often involuntary. All tic behaviors are made worse by stress. They are not present during sleep and may be less apparent during activity.

Motor tics vary from simple, abrupt movements, such as eye blinking, head jerking, or shoulder shrugging, to more complex, purposeful-appearing behaviors, such as facial expressions or gestures of the arms or head. In extreme cases, these movements can be obscene or self-injurious (hitting or biting). Vocal tics can range from simple throat-clearing sounds to more complex vocalizations and speech. At the onset of tic behaviors it may be difficult to know that they are tics. It may not be possible to establish a diagnosis until the full clinical picture has developed over time.

Tics have other characteristics. They are intermittent, not continuous. They vary in time, location, frequency, and amplitude. Some individuals observe that the tic is preceded by an irresistible urge, followed by relief.

The face and neck are the most frequently involved parts of the body, with a descending gradient of frequency from face to feet.

The most common tics include

1) Face and head: grimacing, puckering of forehead, raising eyebrows, blinking eyelids, winking, wrinkling nose, trembling nostrils, twitching mouth, displaying teeth, biting lips and other parts, extruding tongue, protracting lower jaw, nodding, jerking or shaking the head, twisting neck, looking sideways, and head rolling

2) Arms and hands: jerking hands, jerking arms, plucking fingers, writhing fingers, and clenching fists

3) Body and lower extremities: shrugging shoulders; shaking feet, knees, or toes; peculiarities of gait, body writhing, and jumping

4) Respiratory and alimentary: hiccupping, sighing, yawning, snuffing, blowing through nostrils, whistling, inspiration, exaggerated breathing, belching, sucking or smacking sounds, and clearing throat

Tic disorders are classified by the length of time the tics lasts. *Transient tic disorder* is defined as recurrent, repetitive, rapid, purposeless motor movements. The average age of onset is 7 years. The tics last weeks or months then fade away, not to return.

*Chronic motor tic disorder* is defined with the same pattern and timing of tics as noted with transient tic disorder; however, the intensity of the behaviors is consistent over weeks or months. The tics must last for at least 1 year to be considered a chronic motor tic disorder.

*Tourette disorder* is characterized by recurrent, involuntary, repetitive, rapid, purposeless motor tics, and multiple vocal tics. There is a strong family history. Along with motor tics described above, vocal tics are present in about 60% of all cases and include various complicated sounds and words. With patients, there is an irresistible urge to utter obscenities. Vocal tics may be clicks, grunts, yelps, barks, sniffs, coughs, or words.

The pediatrician can and should consider these related disorders if the office assessment suggests a learning, language, and/or motor disability and follow-up studies confirm the diagnosis. Does the child have ADHD? Is there a chronic and pervasive history of an anxiety disorder, depression, intermittent explosive disorder, or obsessive-compulsive disorder? Does the child have a tic disorder? Does the history suggest a bipolar disorder?

Pediatricians can evaluate for and treat ADHD and many cases of tic disorders. If one of the emotional regulatory problems or bipolar disorder is suspected, it might be best for the pediatrician to seek a consultation with and assistance from a mental health professional for further evaluation and treatment.

Often the differential process is complex. For example, the child shows a chronic and pervasive pattern of depression and of problems with anger control. Are these 2 disorders reflective of emotional regulatory problems or the result of bipolar disorder? Sometimes knowing the relevant medical history of a family member aids in diagnosis. Again, when the situation is unclear, it might be best to seek consultation with a mental health professional.

## Conclusion

While preparing this chapter, one of the authors (LBS) was asked to evaluate a 13-year-old girl, Marlene, who had been diagnosed with ADHD. Her medication was not working and she continued to do poorly in school.

When I met with her parents and then with her, I did find a chronic and pervasive history of inattention, manifested by auditory and visual distractibility. She reported that when she was taking her medication (Concerta), she could pay attention but she still did poorly. I did the systems review set of questions described in this book. It became clear that she was struggling with reading comprehension and with written language skills. Formal psychoeducational testing done later confirmed the learning disability.

However, given our knowledge of the pattern of comorbidity described in this chapter, I went through another pattern of clinical assessments. Neither she nor her parents described problems with anxiety or depression. She had no difficulties with anger control. Her parents did not describe behaviors suggestive of obsessive or compulsive problems or of tics.

I met with Marlene. She, too, did not describe problems with anxiety or depression. Toward the end of the diagnostic session I asked about obsessional thoughts. She said that she often worried that she might get sick and vomit. She was terrified of vomiting. She went on to say that she did everything she could to not get sick. She took at least 2 showers a day, often taking 30 or more minutes. She changed her clothes several times a day. Marlene would not use public bathrooms. I then asked about compulsive behaviors. She smiled uncomfortably and told me of her need to count. She counted by twos and could only stop if she was on an even number. If she touched something, she had to touch it an even number of times. Before going to bed she had to check her closet door and the lock on her window 2 or 3 times. I asked if she had ever shared these problems with her parents. She said no. I wondered why and she said that she was too embarrassed.

With her permission, she joined me when I met with her parents to discuss my clinical impressions. She agreed that I could discuss all that we had discussed. I reviewed my impression that she did have ADHD. I introduced the idea of a possible learning disability and discussed the type of studies needed. Then I began to describe Marlene's obsessive and compulsive behaviors. Father was astonished. Mother began to cry. I asked why she was upset. She said, "You know, I have had the same problems since I was a little girl. I thought that they were so strange that I could not tell anyone else. I didn't know anyone else could be like me." Both mother and daughter accepted treatment for their obsessive-compulsive disorder.

Prior to the knowledge provided by statistical studies looking for relationships between one of the disorders in *DSM-IV-TR* and another, the relationships described in this chapter would not have been apparent. Many children were not diagnosed with the related disorders because we did not think to do so.

We used to teach that the side effects of the stimulant medications might include becoming emotionally fragile (anxious or depressed) or might cause angry outbursts. We also thought that these stimulant medications caused tics. Now we know that these new behaviors are reflective of other disorders that are exacerbated, not caused, by the stimulants.

But if you don't look for it, you won't find it. And, if you don't find it, you can't provide treatment. The value of this new knowledge is to remind clinicians that if any one of the disorders on the list is found, it is essential that questions be directed toward clarifying if one or more of the other disorders might also be present. It is equally important to continually be on the lookout for the emergence or unmasking of other disorders over time.

## *Bibliography*

Brown TE, ed. *ADHD Comorbidities. Handbook for ADHD Complications in Children and Adults*. Washington, DC: American Psychiatric Publishing, Inc.; 2009

Carlson GA, Meyer SE. ADHD with mood disorders. In: Brown TE, ed. *ADHD Comorbidities. Handbook for ADHD Complications in Children and Adults*. Washington, DC: American Psychiatric Publishing, Inc.; 2009:97–130

Geller DA, Brown TE. ADHD with obsessive-compulsive disorder. In: Brown TE, ed. *ADHD Comorbidities. Handbook for ADHD Complications in Children and Adults*. Washington, DC: American Psychiatric Publishing, Inc.; 177–188

Newcorn JH, Halperin JM, Miller CJ. ADHD with oppositionality and aggression. In: Brown TE, ed. *ADHD Comorbidities. Handbook for ADHD Complications in Children and Adults*. Washington, DC: American Psychiatric Publishing, Inc.; 157–176

Papolos D, Papolos J. *The Bipolar Child*. 3rd ed. New York, NY: Broadway Books; 2006

Sukhodolsky DG, Scahill L, Leekman JF. ADHD with Tourette syndrome. In: Brown TE, ed. *ADHD Comorbidities. Handbook for ADHD Complications in Children and Adults*. Washington, DC: American Psychiatric Publishing, Inc.; 293–304

Tannock R, Brown TE. ADHD with language and/or learning disorders in children and adolescents. In: Brown TE, ed. *ADHD Comorbidities. Handbook for ADHD Complications in Children and Adults*. Washington, DC: American Psychiatric Publishing, Inc.; 189–232

Tannock T. ADHD with anxiety. In: Brown TE, ed. *ADHD Comorbidities. Handbook for ADHD Complications in Children and Adults*. Washington, DC: American Psychiatric Publishing, Inc.; 131–156

# Chapter 9

# The Related Pragmatic Social Skills Disabilities

For some children, their social skills problems are not secondary to the frustrations and failures resulting from their disabilities. These social skills problems are another reflection of a dysfunctional nervous system. They seem to misread visual cues, such as a look on someone's face or a body stance. They also might misread auditory cues, such as the tone of voice or speed of speech. Often they have equal difficulty understanding how others might read their body language.

As with other neurologically based problems, these social skills problems have a chronic and a pervasive history. They reflect the individual's difficulties reading social cues.

Such pragmatic social skills difficulties may also be seen with children who are on the pervasive developmental disorder spectrum. Often, in these clinical situations, the intensity of the problems is more than that found with children who have learning disabilities. Children with learning disabilities can relate to others around them; however, some of their behaviors may be annoying to others. It will be helpful first to describe normal pragmatic social skills. With this knowledge as a baseline, it will be possible to describe pragmatic social skills disabilities.

- **Facial expressions:** Facial movements and poses communicate emotion. Effective eye contact and the appropriate use of facial expressions, such as smiling, are 2 of the most frequently noted.
- **Postures and gestures:** Hand and arm movements that communicate meaning are called *gestures*; positions of the entire body that convey meaning are called *postures*. Both gestures and postures can convey messages that conflict with spoken words, confusing communication effects.
- **Interpersonal distance (space) and touch:** People have a personal comfort space around them. If a child stands too close to others while talking, that child is violating the rules of personal space. A child who touches others inappropriately either in terms of the location or the intensity of that

contact (eg, hugging) breaks one of the unwritten laws of touch and might cause anger or rejection.

## Auditory Perception

- **Paralanguage:** This term refers to those aspects of sound that communicate emotion and that are used either independently or with words. Examples are intensity and loudness of voice, and whistling and humming a tune.
- **Rhythm and time:** Speech patterns, attitudes, and speed of movement or speech all fall into the category of rhythm. Some children do not correctly perceive that the person's rate and flow of speech is communicating an emotion—annoyance, frustration. Problems may occur when the child's rate and rhythm are faster or slower than expected.
- **Volume:** The loudness or softness of voice communicates emotions. A teacher's loud voice may communicate annoyance; a soft voice may communicate the wish that students be quiet. The child misreads facial movements and expressions that, along with the words said, might communicate how the other person is feeling (anger, frustration, annoyance or smiling, laughing). This child might not understand how his or her expressions or lack of expressions are interpreted (eg, eye contact, smiling, frowning).

## *Pragmatic Social Skills Disabilities*

The literature on pragmatic social skills disabilities is relatively new and growing. The term is descriptive of the problems found. There is no formal diagnostic category for these disabilities within *Diagnostic and Statistical Manual of Mental Disorders, Fourth Edition.*

We can observe nonverbal communication from 2 perspectives. First, does the child correctly read nonverbal social cues while interacting with another? A teacher is standing in front of Billy's desk, looking directly at him. Her face is taut and her voice is loud as she says, "Stop that right now!" Billy looks up surprised. Did Billy pick up the earlier cues that his behavior was upsetting the teacher? Did he observe these cues as they escalated?

The other perspective is whether the child has a concept of how others perceive the nonverbal social cues he or she is communicating. Ellen is too close to her friend, almost in her face. Her voice is loud and she is jumping up and down. Her friend pushes her away and says, "Leave me alone." Ellen is surprised and hurt to be rejected by her friend. Was she aware of her nonverbal communication and how it was perceived by her friend?

Thus pragmatic social skills difficulties may involve difficulties with auditory and/or visual nonverbal communication. The problem could be that the child misreads the social cues coming from others or that the child does not realize the messages his social behaviors are communicating to others.

## Problems With Visual Communication

### Facial Expressions

Can the child recognize a happy face? A sad face? An angry face? A fearful face? Can she present her face with the proper expression for the way she is feeling? A mother is upset with something her daughter is doing and angry that she has not stopped doing it. Her face is stern and communicates anger. Finally, she says, "Jane, you make me so angry." Jane looks up and says, "Why are you angry?" Later, her mother perceives Jane's body language as showing that she is angry. She asks what she is angry about. Jane replies, "I'm not angry."

### Space and Touch

As described earlier, most people have informal space zones of comfort. Who can enter any zone is defined by that zone and is often culturally determined. Studies suggest that there are 4 such zones. The public zone refers to areas identified as not being a part of one's life, such as walking in the street, riding on a bus, or going through a shopping center. There seems to be a certain space needed between a person and others around him or her. Next is the social zone. A person who is known by the individual might enter this zone. The third zone is personal space. People you know very well can enter this space. Depending on culture, friends might shake hands, offer a kiss on the cheek, or give a big hug. The fourth zone is intimate space. This space is reserved for special, significant others: spouse, parent, child.

Some children do not understand or respect concepts of space. They may go up to a stranger and give a hug, or get too close and make others feel uncomfortable.

Touch is related to space. How one touches and the intensity of the touch changes as one moves into the 4 social zones. A child can sit on his mother's lap and snuggle, hug, and kiss. Such behavior may not be appropriate or comfortable if he is sitting on the lap of a certain aunt, a family friend, or a babysitter, depending on the family dynamic. There are certain touch rules or taboos that must be followed.

## Gestures and Postures

Gestures start with learning to wave bye-bye. Other gestures are then added. Think of your hand and arm gestures when you say, "stop," "behave," "come here," or "right now." There is something about the hand position as well as the lower- and upper-arm and shoulder position that communicates the message and the intensity of the message. We have head gestures such as "yes," "no," and "I'm confused." Our total body stance and degree of muscle tone help us communicate through our posture. Nonverbally, we show anger, tension, confusion, and annoyance. How someone leans forward, places their hands on a desk, sits, or walks also communicates messages. Some children have difficulty reading nonverbal visual messages, as well as understanding how others read their actions.

# Problems With Auditory Communication

## Tone of Voice

Some children speak too loudly or they speak with a tone that does not match the emotional message intended. Josh speaks softly as he says, "Shut up! You are making me mad." Alice yells angrily, "Have a good day." So, too, some children misread the tone of voice of the adult or child.

## Rate of Speech

Rapid speech can be irritating to others. Slow speech may suggest insecurity or lack of the knowledge to respond. Slow speech may cause a listener to become impatient.

## Emphasis or Variations in Speech

Variations in volume and word emphasis help the listener understand the meaning of what is being said. Speaking in a monotone can be confusing, causing a listener to perceive the speaker as dull or unresponsive.

## *Treatment for Pragmatic Social Skills Problems*

Secondary social skills problems are best helped by working with the child, family, and school professionals to help the child become more successful in all settings and activities. Pragmatic social skills difficulties are best treated in a specially designed social skills group where pragmatic skills are taught and practiced. At this time such social skills groups are run by mental health professionals.

Pragmatic social skills groups often use a specific curriculum and specific materials. Skills are taught and practiced in a way similar to teaching reading or writing. For example, a series of pictures of faces are shown with the group leader identifying the emotion reflected. The children practice recognizing each face. Later the leader might ask the children to show an angry face or a sad face. The children agree or disagree on the emotion expressed. Still later a child might make a face and the others are asked to determine the emotion being expressed. In this step-by-step, didactic way, each of the pragmatic social skills are introduced and taught.

The pediatrician plays an important role in recognizing that a child might have social problems because of pragmatic social skills difficulties. Parents should be educated about the problems and then directed to a mental health professional who can both help the child and the family address these problems.

## *Bibliography*

Duke MP, Norwicki Jr SI, Martin EA. *Teaching Your Child the Language of Social Success.* Atlanta, GA: Peachtree Press; 1996

Lavoie R. *It's So Much Work to Be Your Friend. Helping the Child with Learning Disabilities Find Social Success.* New York, NY: Touchstone; 2005

Silver LB. *The Misunderstood Child. Understanding and Coping with Your Child's Learning Disabilities.* 4th ed. New York, NY: Three Rivers Press; 2006

# Part III

# Clinical Interventions: The Public School System

# Chapter 10

# The Public School: Laws and Policies

The first major piece of legislation to ensure a free and appropriate education for children with disabilities was the Rehabilitation Act of 1973, specifically Section 504 of the law. This law provided that "no otherwise qualified individual with a disability…be excluded from participation in, be denied the benefits of, or be subjected to discrimination under any program or activity receiving Federal financial assistance." Section 504 of this law refers to educational settings. School systems today refer to a "504 plan" to describe accommodations and possible services for students with disabilities.

The major piece of legislation focused on the need to educate all students, including those with disabilities was the Education for All handicapped Children Act of 1975 (Public Law 94-142). It provided a number of unprecedented mandates, such as a free appropriate public education (FAPE), procedural rights, due process, and education in the least-restricted environment. This single piece of legislation changed forever the process by which students with disabilities received education in public schools. This law has been reauthorized many times (1986, 1990, 1997, 2004), each time expanding and refining the practices, policies, and procedures that govern the inclusion of students with disabilities in our schools.

The revisions of 1986 expanded the ages covered to include from birth through age 21. Infants and toddlers programs (covering birth–36 months) were added to the existing early intervention programs for ages 3 to 5 (Child Find). In 1998, in keeping with the concept of political correctness, the name of the law was changed from Education for All Handicapped Children to Individuals with Disabilities Education Act, or IDEA. In 2004 the concept of response to intervention (RTI) was included. This concept will be discussed in detail later in this chapter.

# Individuals with Disabilities Education Act

The IDEA is the federal legislation for special education services in the United States. It protects the rights of individuals with disabilities and regulates how states and public agencies provide special education and related services to these individuals.

The IDEA identifies 14 different categories of disabilities. Children with these disabilities receive special educational services, described as "specially designed instruction designed to meet the unique needs of a child with a disability." The 14 categories are mental retardation, hearing impaired, deafness, speech or language impairment, visual impairment, emotional disturbance, orthopedic impaired, other health impaired, specific learning disabilities, multiple disabilities, deaf-blindness, traumatic brain injury, autism, and developmental delay (applies to children ages 3–5 only). There are 5 major provisions found in IDEA (Box 10-1).

Remember that Section 504 of the Rehabilitation Act is a civil rights law that prohibits discrimination against individuals who meet the definition of having a disability due to a physical or mental impairment that substantially limits a major life activity. Section 504 guarantees that a child with a disability has equal access to an appropriate education. Unlike IDEA, Section 504 does not require the school to provide a specific plan (an individualized education program [IEP]) to meet a child's specific educational needs. The child may, however, receive accommodations and modifications to their educational needs.

Thus an IEP must define both services and accommodations for the individual with a disability. Section 504 plans need only identify necessary accommodations. (The details of an IEP will be discussed later.) In many school systems, if a child does not meet the criteria listed for establishing a specific disability and, thus, cannot be considered under IDEA, the school professionals might establish a 504 plan. Under this plan, it is possible to provide some services along with the accommodations. By doing this, it is possible to provide all services and programs that would be in an IEP by including them in the 504 plan.

Attention-deficit/hyperactivity disorder (ADHD) is not one of the disabilities listed in IDEA. Thus a child cannot be serviced under this law for this disability. Some school systems will classify the child with a disability as "other health impaired" under this law. By doing this, an IEP can be

---

### Box 10-1. Major Provisions in IDEA

1. *Screening and Identification:* School systems must be alert to students who show difficulties and screen to determine if further assessments are necessary. Procedures are established to identify children in need of special education services and possibly placement in a special education program. A significant feature of this provision is Child Find. This is the process of public awareness, screening, and evaluation designed to identify and to refer as early as possible young children with disabilities and their families who are in need of early intervention services or preschool special education services.

2. *Nondiscriminatory Evaluation:* This second provision involves ensuring that evaluations are nondiscriminatory. That is, the selection and administration of tests should not be racially or culturally biased. Guidelines provide specific requirements about how evaluations should be conducted. Tests used must be valid for the purpose used. The evaluators must be knowledgeable and trained to use the test material. A variety of instruments and procedures must be used, and the test results must accurately reflect the student's aptitude or achievement level rather than reflect only on the student's disabilities.

3. *FAPE and LRE:* The child with a disability must be provided a free appropriate public education (FAPE) in the least-restrictive environment (LRE).

4. *Procedural Safeguards:* Procedural safeguards must be in place to protect the rights of children with disabilities and their parents. These safeguards include protection in notification of procedures to the parents, due process hearings, mediation, and an appeals process.

5. *Due Process:* The final provision of IDEA is that individuals with disabilities and their families are guaranteed the right of due process as established by Amendment XIV of the US Constitution. The IDEA identifies specific requirements for both families and schools and provides impartial hearings when a disagreement occurs involving the identification, evaluation, placement, or service delivery for an individual with a disability.

---

written. Other school systems will use the diagnosis of ADHD and prepare a 504 plan.

## The Process of Identifying and Defining Needs

If the classroom teacher and other school professionals are concerned about a child, the principal will establish a meeting between the child's parents, the teacher, and all relevant professionals. At this meeting, all observations and findings are presented to the parents. If further studies are needed to clarify the problems, the child's parents must agree and sign a release permitting such studies.

Parents might also initiate such a meeting by giving the principal a letter requesting that the classroom teacher, school professionals, and the principal meet to discuss their concerns about their child. (Schools are not required to honor verbal requests.) Once the principal receives this letter, the meeting must be called. It is during this process that a report or letter from the child's pediatrician stating concerns about the child is most valuable. During this exploratory meeting, all concerns are discussed. Parents might request further formal studies to clarify why their child is having difficulty. Some parents might have their child evaluated privately prior to this meeting. The formal psychoeducational, speech and language, occupational therapy, or other studies are provided to the principal so that all attending the meeting can read them in advance.

After all studies have been completed or, if done privately, all such testing has been accepted by the school system, a second-level meeting is called. This meeting is often called an *IEP meeting*. The school professionals present the findings of their studies. Using the criteria established for their school system, they review 3 issues. Each issue must be agreed on by both the school professionals and the parents before they can be acted on.

1) Does the child have a disability based on the definition for that disability under IDEA, as used by the school system?
2) If it is agreed that the child has a disability, what specific services will be needed to address this disability?
3) Given the services needed, in what setting will these services be provided (general education classroom, general education classroom with pullout times to provide specific services, a special education program)?

Once each of these issues is agreed on by the school professionals and the parents, a contract is written defining specifically what services and accommodations will be provided, where and for how long each service will be provided, and how progress will be measured. This contract is an IEP. Once the school administrator and the parents sign this IEP, it is implemented. It is expected that parents and professionals will meet annually to review the IEP and make any modifications necessary.

If the school professionals conclude that the child does not meet the criteria to be identified as having a disability, no IEP will be prepared. These professionals might present a 504 plan as an alternative. As noted previously, this plan defines what accommodations will be provided the child. The provision of services is not required; however, some school systems will identify services along with the accommodations.

Parents must be involved at each step of this process, from the initial meeting to the finalization of decisions and later modifications. Parents must be informed of their right to appeal and the process for appealing.

A pediatrician should also be aware of several other services that might be included in the IEP, the extended school year (ESY), transition planning, and related services. A parent's request for each is strengthened by a letter from the child's pediatrician.

## Extended School Year

The ESY services are individualized instructional programs for students with disabilities that are provided beyond the length of the regular school year. These programs usually occur during the summer when school is not in session. An ESY is provided for students with disabilities or significantly interfering behaviors when they require continuous instruction or services to prevent regression or loss of skills acquired during the school year. The ESY services may also be provided when skills are emerging and continuous instruction or support is necessary for full skill acquisition.

## Transition Plan

A transition plan is a set of activities developed for a student with a disability to ensure that their academic and functional progress helps prepare them for movement from school to post-school activities. Postsecondary school activities may include postsecondary education, vocational education, employment (including supported employment), continuing and adult education, adult services, independent living, or community participation. These transition plans are usually initiated at age 14. By age 16, specific transition services and activities should be included, along with the early phases of identification and coordination of postsecondary services. The transition plan is based on the individual child's needs, strengths, and interests and may include classroom-based instruction, community experiences, vocational training, and functional daily living skills.

## Response to the Intervention Model of Assessment

The 2004 reauthorization of IDEA established the goal of having "highly qualified instructors" to teach children with disabilities and the expectation that "scientific research-based instructions" would be used. In an effort to shift from formal testing to establish the diagnosis of a learning disability, a new model of assessment was encouraged if not expected to be used. This is the RTI model. Core to its success is having highly qualified instructors who use scientific research-based instructions. Many professionals see promise in using this new model for assessment. However, concern is expressed about the application of this approach for assessment before either appropriately trained teachers or available researched interventions are available. Some express concern about the lack of clarity regarding how much time might be spent at each level of intervention before the next level should be started. The fear is that students may not receive adequate interventions, delaying the time it takes to establish the reasons for the academic difficulties and to provide the appropriate help. The RTI model has 3 phases of intervention.

- Phase 1: If a student is not making progress, he or she is identified and the classroom teacher tries additional instructional materials to help the student move ahead. (Again, the concern with using RTI is that not all general education teachers are trained to try additional instructional materials and that there are not yet adequate scientific research-based methods of instruction available.)
- Phase 2: If the student makes limited progress during Phase 1, a consultant is assigned to work with the general education teacher and the student. (Given the reductions in funding and staffing within special education, there is concern that there will not be enough highly qualified special education teachers to perform this role.)
- Phase 3: The RTI model as described in the 2004 revision of IDEA suggests that if the student does not make progress within Phase 2, an IEP should be prepared and the student moved into a special education program.

Many professionals who work with students with disabilities express concern with this approach. Unless some series of testing is done, how will anyone know the reasons for the student's difficulties? This student might have problems because of poor previous education or cultural, bilingual, social, or environmental factors. Or he or she might have problems because of their level of intellectual functioning, learning disabilities, or another psychiatric disorder (eg, autism, another pervasive developmental disorder, a psychotic disorder). How can an IEP be prepared without knowing the factors contributing to the student's difficulties? A second concern is that without such an assessment, each student could only be placed in a class based on the severity of problems. Rather than services for students with learning, language, motor, or other disabilities, programs might only be identified as "mild," "moderate," or "severe." The mix of students in each class might cover all of the possibilities noted above. Such a placement would be a major challenge for the teaching staff and would make it more than difficult to individualize the instruction to the specific needs of each student.

At the time this book was prepared, the RTI model was in effect in many school systems. If your patient is in a program that does not do an assessment between Phase 2 and Phase 3 to clarify the reasons for the child's difficulties prior to writing an IEP, it is important that you educate parents and support the need to request such assessments. *Parents should know that by law they can request formal testing at any time.*

## Related Services

Students with disabilities are often at risk for mental health problems. Schools often provide support through a variety of what are called *related services.* Mental health services in a school setting may be delivered in a number of ways. The most common approaches for delivery of these services involve individual and/or group therapy services. Individual therapy services are typically delivered by a licensed mental health service provider (social worker, school psychologists, counselor). Group therapy services in special education focus on the development of the skills a student requires to be successful in the classroom and, thus, benefit from education. These services might involve social skills development, recreational groups, or groups focused on specific deficit areas, such as communication, behavior, managing emotions, cooperative learning, and/or coping strategies.

# *The Appeal Process*

If parents are not happy with the conclusions the school professionals reach, they have 2 options for appealing these decisions. They might choose a mediator to resolve the differences between what they believe is needed and what the school professionals are recommending, or they might initiate a due process hearing.

## Mediation

Mediation is the process of having an impartial trained person, called a *mediator,* try to help parents and the school system reach an agreement about their child's special education program and services. Mediation is more informal than a due process hearing. Both the parents and the school system have to agree in order for mediation to occur. If agreement is reached, it will be put in writing. If no agreement is reached, the mediation discussion will remain confidential and cannot be used in any subsequent due process hearing. If a school system fails to implement a mediation agreement, a parent can go to court to enforce the agreement.

If a parent wishes to request mediation, this request must be in writing. A copy of the request is sent to the school system and to the state Department of Health Office of Administrative Hearings. Once requested, the mediation session should occur within 20 calendar days from the date received.

## Due Process Hearings

A due process hearing is a formal way to resolve a dispute between parents and the school system about the child's education program. An administrative law judge, appointed through the state Office of Administrative Hearings, runs the hearing.

During the IEP process, the school system retains control over every decision. By requesting a hearing, the parent can take this decision-making control away from the school system. The hearing officer will then make the decision. The hearing can address any issue related to the provision of special education and related services for a child.

# *Students in Special Education*

Students receiving special education services are protected from specific disciplinary procedures under IDEA. All too often, students receiving special education services are overrepresented in the number of students suspended or expelled from school. The requirements within IDEA attempt to strike a fair balance between effective discipline and providing appropriate supports for students with disabilities. These regulations do not prevent school officials from maintaining a safe school environment conducive to learning. It is recognized that inappropriate behaviors cannot interfere with the education of others or disrupt the education process. There are 2 main categories of disciplinary action covered by IDEA: suspension and expulsion.

## Suspension

Suspension from school is characterized as the temporary removal of a student from a school setting for disciplinary reasons. The specific regulations provided by IDEA for disciplinary procedures limit schools to 10 cumulative days of suspension per year for students in special education. Schools are not required to provide special education services during the first 10 days of a suspension. Suspensions up to 10 days can occur against parental approval if discipline procedures are applied consistently to all students. Suspensions longer than 10 days constitute a change in placement and trigger the procedural protections of IDEA. Students may have protection under IDEA only if they are currently receiving special education services or have been referred for special education services, and the school had knowledge of the disability.

*In-school suspension* is defined as the expulsion within the school building of a student from general education activities for disciplinary reasons. In-school suspension is often used by schools as a consequence for behaviors that do not reach the level of severity requiring out-of-school suspension or expulsion. In-school suspensions are counted as part of the cumulative 10 days of suspension per year for special education students.

*Alternative education settings* are placements created for specific disciplinary violations. Students engaging in drug/alcohol use or bringing in weapons to school are subject to discipline regardless of disability. If the IEP and placement of a student with a disability are determined to be appropriate, the student is subject to the same disciplinary actions as his or her nondisabled peers. For violations requiring such an alternative education setting, a placement will be provided for up to 45 days. Then a reevaluation is necessary to determine future placement.

## Expulsion

An expulsion for a student is characterized as the permanent removal of a student from the educational setting. Students with disabilities are afforded specific protections regarding expulsion. Following the recommendation for expulsion of a student receiving special education services, the IEP team must meet for a "manifestation determination." That is, is there a relationship between the student's behavior subject to discipline and the student's disability. If a student's suspension exceeds 10 days or if a recommendation for expulsion is made by the school, a manifestation determination meeting must take place within 10 days of the date of disciplinary action.

Critical for this manifestation determination is to clarify if any of the following are true: (1) the IEP or placement was inappropriate or the IEP was not being implemented, including appropriate behavior intervention strategies; (2) the child does not have the capacity to understand the consequences of his or her behavior due to the disability; (3) the child's disability prevented his or her ability to control behaviors; or (4) the child is unable to conform to the schools rules due to the disability.

During proceedings to determine manifestation, the student is either suspended, as long as 10 days have not passed, or he or she must remain in current placement until the question is resolved. If parents disagree with the outcome of this manifestation meeting, they may initiate due process proceedings.

## Conclusion

Education laws are clear. They set guidelines for evaluating and working with students who have special needs. These services are available from birth through the end of the 21st birthday. It is important that pediatricians understand these laws so that they can advise parents of their rights within the school system.

# Bibliography

Latham PS, Latham PH, Mandelawitz M. *Special Education Law*. Washington, DC: JKL Communications; 2008

Wright PWD, Wright PD. *Wrightslaw: Special Education Law*. Hartfield, VA: Harbor House Law Press; 2008

# Chapter 11

# The Public School: Assessment and Intervention

When the result of your office screening assessment suggests that the reason your patient is struggling in school is a possible learning disability, a full assessment should be done to confirm whether your clinical impression is correct. And, if the child has a learning disability, it is essential that he or she receive the necessary accommodations and services. The pediatrician's participation in the referral and assessment process is essential to ensuring a child's success.

This chapter focuses on the full process mentioned in Chapter 10: from the initial request to the screening process, the assessment process, and the decision-making process. The types of interventions that are used within the public school system will also be discussed. With each of these steps, the pediatrician's input and information is essential. It is important that the pediatrician understand the school system's approach to assessment and management of children with special needs. In this way they can help empower the parents to be the best advocate for their child.

## Assessment Overview

The formal assessment process might start with a psychoeducational or a neuropsychological evaluation. The psychoeducational evaluation focuses on the brain processing abilities necessary for learning and identifies strengths and weaknesses. The psychoeducational evaluation also evaluates for attentional and emotional problems. The neuropsychological evaluation includes all studies within a psychoeducational evaluation as well as other studies focused on broader brain functions. If there is clinical evidence to suggest a problem, assessment by a speech-language pathologist, occupational therapist, or other specialist should be conducted.

All necessary studies should be done by public school professionals if possible. The cost for a privately conducted psychoeducational evaluation ranges from $2,000 to $3,000 or more. Should further speech-language or occupational therapy evaluations also be needed, the cost increases. It is probable that the family's health insurance plan would cover little, if any, of the costs of private testing.

Exceptions do exist if there are concerns about the risk of possible brain damage (eg, lead poisoning, head injury). A neuropsychological assessment can be requested that will provide all of the information in a psychoeducational assessment plus additional studies of brain function/dysfunction. Sometimes a letter from the child's pediatrician stressing that these studies are essential to their finalizing their medical treatment plan may facilitate coverage for part or all of the assessments.

Example: "Billy Jones is under my *medical* care. He has neurologically based difficulties with both receptive and expressive language tasks. It is *medically necessary* for him to have a comprehensive speech and language evaluation to assist me in finalizing my *medical treatment plan*. These studies have been ordered by me and the results will be reviewed and used by me."

Under IDEA, the public school system must provide screening, assessment and, when needed, intervention services. As discussed in Chapter 10, the public school system must provide assessment and intervention services for children ages 3 and up. Children in the zero to 3 age group are covered by the Infants and Toddlers Program, as defined by Part H of IDEA. When necessary, services can be provided until the end of the 21st birthday. To initiate such a request for evaluation, parents must start with the principal of their local public school. (If a parent does not know which school to go to, they can call their central public school office and ask for the Child Find number.) If their child is younger than 5 or goes to a private school, parents can still initiate the request with the principal of their local public school.

## *The Public School System*

Public schools have administrative, general education, and special education professionals who provide services within the general education setting, the special education programs or, when needed, in private programs. The types of services provided are based on the specific needs of each child.

## School Personnel

The administrative head of each school is the principal, and all programs are under this professional's guidance and supervision. Any request for assessment or for services must be presented in writing to the principal. He or she will then schedule all meetings and often chairs the meetings.

Each school should have a team of specialists. (In many areas, this group is called the *child study team.*) Some programs have access to other specific specialist from the broader school system. The school psychologist, often a master's level or a PhD/PsyD, usually observes a child, works with a teacher on managing classroom behaviors, and/or performs the psychological part of a psychoeducational evaluation. Many schools also have a school counselor who is available to make observations or provide psychological supportive services. A special education consultant trained in the area of learning disabilities can perform the educational part of the psychoeducational evaluation, provide specific interventions, and coordinate the services needed by a child. A speech-language therapist and an occupational therapist should be available at each school to screen and, when needed, to assess a child suspected of having a language and/or a motor problem.

## School Settings

The primary classrooms and programs within the public school are for students with no special needs, referred to as *general education.* Classrooms and programs for students with special needs are referred to as *special education.* Services for students with learning disabilities might be provided in either setting.

If the child is in a general education classroom and receives specific services provided by a specialist who comes into the classroom, the intervention is referred to as *mainstreaming* or *inclusion.* Should the child leave the general education classroom during specific times of specific days to receive special education services within the special education programs, the intervention is referred to as a *pullout program.* Some children might spend part or all of the day in a special education program. A few might be in a separate school providing comprehensive special education services. This self-contained school might be part of the public school system or a private special education school.

## Types of Services

The child with learning disabilities needs specific interventions depending on the types of disabilities and the effect these disabilities have on the learning process. *Remedial interventions* focus on minimizing or correcting the underlying processing disorders. As an example, if a child is having difficulty learning to read because of weak phonological skills, phonological training will facilitate learning to read. For students who have learning disabilities that are not fully addressed by remedial interventions, *compensatory strategies* are necessary. For example, a child who has difficulty retrieving and organizing information that must be written would be taught strategies to facilitate those processes.

*Webbing* is an example of a compensatory strategy. Before trying to write, the student would put all of his thoughts about a topic on a page, preferably using key words. The student then is taught how to identify the most important ideas and circle each. The remaining thoughts are circled and lines are drawn to connect words to the major word that it relates to. Eventually this webbing of thoughts can be made into an outline. Once outlined and organized, the student begins to write. Because remedial or compensatory strategies take extra time, students with learning disabilities often need appropriate accommodations. Such accommodations include more time on tests or classroom assignments, a note taker, a copy of material placed on the board, organizational assistance, permission to use a calculator or a computer in class, or textbooks and other necessary materials on tape.

Remedial and compensatory strategies are provided by specially trained professionals, which may include a special education specialist, a remedial reading teacher, a speech-language therapist, and/or an occupational therapist. It is not acceptable for a classroom aide or a volunteer to be assigned to provide the services of these professionals. Accommodations are designed to maximize the student's strengths while accommodating for the weaknesses. These interventions are used in the general education classroom and provided by the general education teacher. To carry out these accommodations requires the teacher's knowledge and understanding of the child's abilities and disabilities and the teacher's sensitivity to helping.

# Initiating the Assessment Process

Parents initiate the assessment process by giving the principal a letter requesting that their child be evaluated. This letter should describe the parents' concerns and any information from the classroom teacher or from formal or informal testing. Parents should keep a copy of the letter and all other correspondence for their records. Copies of any privately conducted formal studies should be attached to the letter. As has been stated repeatedly, a letter from the pediatrician supporting the need for such an assessment is important. Also key is a report of the most recent physical evaluation, noting that there are no health problems or identifying any existing health problems. Parents need to know that any request to the principal must be in writing. As noted earlier, federal law states that if a parent requests such an assessment in writing, the school administrator must call a meeting within 10 calendar days. If the request is verbal, the principal should respond in a timely way but does not have to do so.

## The Initial Meeting

The principal or his or her designee will review the information provided, go over all school records or other information, and speak with the classroom teacher. A meeting is scheduled with all relevant school personnel and the parents. At the initial meeting, all relevant materials are discussed and the parents have an opportunity to discuss their concerns. Some parents will bring an educational advocate with them.

If testing was done privately, the team must review the data. The team has 2 options: (1) accept the private reports and enter them into their records (the school system cannot reject private evaluations without justification) or (2) do comparable testing that shows different results and use their reports instead of the private testing. If no prior testing has been done, it may be agreed that formal testing is needed. If so, the types of tests planned are discussed and parents are asked to give permission for such studies. The school team might recommend that further observations be made or informal help be provided. If the school system prefers the response to intervention model (see Chapter 10), this approach will be started. A date for a future meeting is set to review testing and progress, or the school team might disagree with the parents and decide nothing needs to be done.

Regardless of the choice, at the end of this first meeting, parents *must* agree with the decisions reached or state their disagreement. They should remember that they have the right to appeal the decision and, if they do, an appeal process *must* be initiated by the school administration.

## Follow-up Meetings

Once the formal testing is done or the observations and informal interventions have been tried, the principal will call a second meeting of the team with the parents. If the testing supports the diagnosis of a learning disability, a proposed plan of action is presented. If everyone remains concerned about the child but no firm data to support the diagnosis are established, the team might propose to continue to support the student and meet again at a future date. Or, the principal or designated head of the team may conclude that no further actions are needed. Again, parents can appeal the decision if they do not agree.

## Action Plan

If the team agrees that there is a disability, a formal plan of action is presented to the parents. The plan may focus on how the school will accommodate for the problems by preparing a 504 plan (discussed in Chapter 10) or the team might agree that both accommodations and specific interventions are needed and an individualized education program (IEP) is presented for consideration (also discussed in Chapter 10). The 504 plan identifies the disability to be addressed and notes the accommodations to be provided. The IEP is more detailed. No actions can be taken on any proposed plans unless parents agree. If there is disagreement, parents can request mediation or initiate an appeal process.

The IEP defines 3 specific issues: (1) the disabilities are identified as defined in IDEA and noted; (2) the specific services to be provided for each disability are listed with reference points on how progress will be measured; and (3) if necessary, a specific placement is clarified. For example, the child might need to be in a special education program part or full time and the nearest such program might be in another school. Thus the student would need to change schools. Each of these 3 specific issues—diagnosis, services, place where services will be provided—must be agreed on by parents before they can be initiated.

Services recommended to the parents may also include transportation, speech therapy, audiological programs, physical therapy, occupational therapy, therapeutic recreation, psychological services, social work services, and any other necessary help. Here, too, parents must understand why these services are important and agree to each.

If a 504 plan or an IEP is initiated, the principal or the coordinator of special education services for the school will schedule follow-up meetings as needed. At the end of each school year, the plans are reviewed and may be continued into the next year, modified, or dropped. Some parents express fear about having an IEP. They are concerned that an IEP will be in their child's records for life and that their child will be labeled. It is helpful to explain that the IEP is reviewed each year and is continued or discontinued based on need.

## The Assessment Process

Because the testing methods are comparable, and the data are based on age and grade norms, the scores will be the same. The results of formal testing done by the school system should be as accurate as testing done by private professionals. However, the interpretation of the results may be different. Some school systems have guidelines that may result in the same test results being interpreted by a private professional as supporting the diagnosis of a learning disability, whereas a school professional would see the results as not supporting the diagnosis. For example, the private assessment might show a discrepancy between the child's ability and performance and conclude that the child has a learning disability. However, the child's school system might require a greater degree of discrepancy between the child's abilities and performance before the term *learning disability* can be used.

This difference in how each school system defines a disability is important to understand. Education law defines a learning disability as a discrepancy between what would be considered age- and grade-appropriate abilities and the abilities/disabilities a particular child shows. That is, administrative guidelines might create exclusionary factors, such as how far behind a child has to be to meet the criteria for having a learning disability. Schools often use the concept of the extent a child must be behind (discrepancy between grade expectation and level shown by testing). A child might be 1 year behind; however, the school requires that the child be 1½ or 2 years behind to qualify for services.

Unfortunately, this discrepancy model is a "wait to fail" model. For example, at the end of second grade a child's reading and writing skills might be at the early first-grade level. However, the child might not meet the discrepancy formula for that school. He or she would have to fail third grade before being far enough behind to qualify for identification and services. By then the child is further behind and has a year or more of frustration and failure. These experiences have a negative impact on the child and on his or her level of frustration, as well as on self-esteem and self-image.

## The Psychoeducational Evaluation

The primary purpose of the psychoeducational evaluation is to identify a child's areas of learning abilities and, if present, any areas of learning weaknesses or disabilities. The results also should clarify the best interventions to address the weaknesses or disabilities and the types of school settings and programs that will maximize the student's ability to overcome, compensate for, and/or accommodate for these disabilities.

The psychoeducational assessment consists of 3 sets of studies: (1) level of intellectual ability; (2) level of achievement in all expected areas of academic skills; and (3) profile of processing skill strengths and weaknesses in all aspects of receiving, processing, storing and then retrieving, and expressing information both through visual input–motor output pathways and listening–verbally expressing pathways (Box 11-1).

---

**Box 11-1. Processing Pathways**

| | |
|---|---|
| **Input:** | Visual perception |
| | Auditory perception |
| **Integration:** | Sequencing |
| | Abstraction |
| **Organization Memory:** | Working memory |
| | Short-term memory |
| | Long-term memory |
| **Output:** | Language output |
| | Motor output |

---

# Assessment of Intelligence

Intelligence tests are designed to be as culturally and linguistically sensitive to different ethnic groups as possible. If a standard test is seen as biased, other methods of assessment should be used. The most frequently used test of intellectual ability is one of the Wechsler intelligence tests. The Wechsler tests cover each age group.

- The Wechsler Pre-School and Primary Scale of Intelligence (WPPSI) (ages 4–6½)
- The Wechsler Intelligence Scale for Children (WISC) (ages 6–16)
- The Wechsler Adult Intelligence Scale (WAIS) (age ≥17)

Each test battery is timed so that a standardized score, based on national standards for the individual's age, can be used to assess where each individual is compared with where he or she should be.

Each of these test batteries consists of specific subtests, each measuring a specific skill or ability. Six of these subtests measure the ability to receive information verbally and respond orally and represent the individual's verbal IQ. Six of these subtests measure the ability to receive information visually and respond using motor skills and represent the individual's performance IQ. Each of these subtests receives a score from 1 to 19.

If an individual has no apparent processing problems, the scores for the subtest will be very similar. For example, if the child is of average intellectual ability, each of the subtests might be between 8 and 12; of superior ability, each of the subtests might be between 15 and 19; and if of below average ability, each of the subtests might be between 7 and 9 or lower. If a child has processing problems, the performance of each of the subtests that requires processing information using these areas of weakness will be affected. Thus the subtest scores will be scattered, possibly ranging 7 to 9 to 12 to 15. This wide discrepancy in subtest scores results in a wide discrepancy between the verbal and performance IQ.

The most frequently used test for school-aged children is the fourth edition of the WISC (WISC-IV), and assesses specific clusters of skills.

- *Verbal Comprehension Index*
  - Information. The examiner orally asks a series of questions about general topics.
  - Similarities. The examiner orally presents a series of pairs of words. The child explains the similarity of the objects.
  - Vocabulary
  - Comprehension. This is a series of orally presented questions. Formulating the answer requires the child to solve everyday problems or to understand social rules and concepts.
  - Information and word reasoning (supplemental). This is a new subtest in WISC-IV that measures inductive verbal reasoning by asking the child to identify a concept described in a series of clues.
- *Perceptual Reasoning Index*
  - Block design. This test consists of a set of modeled or printed 2-dimensional geometric patterns. The child replicates the patterns using 2-colored cubes.
  - Picture concepts. This is a set of colorful pictures presented in a mixed-up order; the child rearranges the pictures into a logical story sequence.
  - Matrix reasoning. This new subtest assesses nonverbal fluid reasoning by having the child select the missing picture or design from an incomplete visual matrix.
  - Picture completion (supplemental). This test consists of a set of colorful pictures of common objects and scenes, each of which is missing an important part. The child identifies the missing part.
- *Working Memory Index*
  - Digit span. This is a series of orally presented number sequences. The child must repeat verbatim the number sequences for digits forward and in reverse order.
  - Letter-number sequencing
  - Arithmetic (supplemental). This is a series of verbally presented arithmetic problems.

- *Processing Speed Index*
  - Coding and symbol search. This test consists of a series of simple shapes or numbers, each paired with a simple symbol. The child is required to draw the symbol in its corresponding shape or under its corresponding number according to a key.
  - Cancellation (supplemental)

Children with learning disabilities may do well on subtests where their problems do not interfere, and their scores in these areas would suggest their intellectual potential. These same children may not do as well on subtests that demand performance in their areas of disability. Often they reflect how the child is performing in the classroom. These scores may not reflect the child's true intellectual potential.

The results of a WISC-IV assessment on 12-year-old Tom illustrates how the subtest scores clarify the possible reasons for a learning processing problem. Tom has good language skills, including receptive and expressive language abilities. However, he is known to have difficulties with tasks that require visual input and motor output.

The results of a WISC-IV assessment were

| | |
|---|---|
| Verbal comprehension | 128 |
| Perceptual reasoning | 80 |
| Working memory | 90 |
| Processing speed | 100 |
| Full scale | 99 |

To say that Tom is of average intelligence, based on his full scale IQ score, is misleading and incorrect. What might be said is that he shows evidence of superior intelligence based on those subtest scores where he has no apparent disabilities: his verbal skills. When he does tasks that reflect his areas of weakness, he performs at the average or below average level. He is bright but frustrated in school because of this discrepancy between his abilities and disabilities. Added to his frustration is that he probably knows the information taught in school but he is not asked to demonstrate it using his verbal skills. He is graded on what he can produce on paper.

Let's look at the specific subtest scores to illustrate how to understand each score and what the overall results suggest. A subtest score of 10 is average. Scores range from 1 to 19.

### TOM'S VERBAL COMPREHENSION SUBTEST SCORES

| Test | Score | Possible Meaning of Score |
|------|-------|---------------------------|
| Similarities | 15 | Suggests a child of superior intelligence with good reasoning and abstraction abilities |
| Vocabulary | 16 | Suggests a child of superior intelligence who is learning through school and general life experiences |
| Comprehension | 14 | Suggests a child of high average to superior intelligence |
| Information | 15 | Suggests a child of superior intelligence who is learning through school and general life experiences |
| Word reasoning | 13 | Suggests a child of high average ability in verbal reasoning |

### TOM'S PERCEPTUAL REASONING SCORES

| Test | Score | Possible Meaning of Score |
|------|-------|---------------------------|
| Block design | 7 | This low score probably reflects his visual perception, visual memory, and visual motor difficulties plus the anxiety of a timed test. |
| Picture concepts | 8 | This low average score suggests that his visual perception and visual motor disabilities interfered with the test. |
| Matrix reasoning | 8 | This low average score suggests that his visual perception disabilities made it difficult to see a picture/concept and recognize what is missing. |
| Picture completion | 8 | This low average score suggests that his visual perception and visual motor disabilities interfered with the task. |

### TOM'S WORKING MEMORY SUBTEST SCORES

| Test | Score | Possible Meaning of Score |
|---|---|---|
| Digit span | 9 | This average score suggests that his ability to hold onto verbally given numbers was difficult for his intellectual potential. |
| Letter-number sequencing | 9 | This average score suggests that his ability to hold onto visually provided numbers and letters was difficult for his intellectual potential. |
| Arithmetic | 9 | This average score suggests that the level of math he understood and could produce in writing was below what would be expected for his ability. |

### TOM'S PROCESSING SPEED SUBTEST SCORES

| Test | Score | Possible Meaning of Score |
|---|---|---|
| Coding | 8 | This low score reflects his difficulties with visual perception, visual memory, and visual motor tasks plus possibly the impact of anxiety because the test is timed. |
| Symbol search | 10 | This score suggests that when he must use visual perception and visual memory, his abilities are average but below expected performance. |

## Assessment of Achievement Level

Once the intellectual assessment is measured, it is necessary to compare its level with true performance to determine whether the student is achieving or underachieving. Standardized achievement tests are given to measure how a child is performing in specific academic skill areas: reading, writing, and math. The results may be presented either in terms of grade-level performance or in terms of percentile levels for age and grade. The most frequently used test of achievement is the Woodcock-Johnson Psychoeducational Battery. This battery of tests comprises 2 parts: the Woodcock-Johnson

Tests of Achievement (measures individual's skill levels) and the Woodcock-Johnson Tests of Cognitive Abilities (measures individual's ability to apply skills to do specific cognitive tasks).

## Woodcock-Johnson Tests of Achievement

The reading assessment measures the ability to decode familiar and new words as well as nonsense words. Next, there is an assessment of reading comprehension. Finally, there is an assessment of the ability to retain the information and to use this information to answer questions in writing. The writing tasks measure the ability to write, including spelling, grammar, punctuation, and capitalization. The student is also asked to produce a written response to a task. The assessment measures content, organization of information, and quality of language used.

Math tasks measure basic math knowledge as well as knowledge of math skills for each grade level. The child is asked to apply known math skills to new tasks.

A general knowledge section measures the level of general knowledge acquired for each grade level as well as knowledge learned elsewhere.

## Woodcock-Johnson Tests of Cognitive Abilities

This battery of tests assesses for long-term retrieval of information, visual-spatial thinking, phonemic awareness, auditory processing, cognitive fluency, fluid reasoning, and processing speed. The purpose is to identify areas of processing strengths and areas of processing weaknesses and/or deficits.

# *Neuropsychological Evaluation*

As noted earlier, if there is concern about brain function versus brain dysfunction going beyond the specific issues related to learning, a neuropsychological assessment is indicated. These studies will evaluate all areas of the brain and all aspects of brain function.

Psychoeducational assessments focus primarily on the demands of the classroom situation. The results are normally interpreted primarily from a level of performance perspective. The neuropsychological evaluation assesses the level of performance where the results are compared with the child's level of achievement as compared with age or grade-level peers.

A neuropsychological evaluation looks at cognitive functioning but also at motor and sensory-perceptual functioning and memory. For each of these assessments, comparisons are made on the 2 sides of the body with identical tasks to determine if they reveal lateralized disparities.

If cerebral dysfunctions are noted, the neuropsychological assessment attempts to determine how these problems might impact on the individual's day to day functioning in their routine environments. The results also assess how an individual approaches problem-solving, noting areas of strength or weakness.

Given the more extensive studies done within a neuropsychological evaluation, the cost is significantly more than for a psychoeducational evaluation. School systems will only do a psychoeducational evaluation. Thus parents must decide if the additional data provided by a neuropsychological evaluation are worth the added cost.

## Other Assessments

As noted previously, a medical evaluation by the child's pediatrician is usually necessary. The pediatrician will be asked to provide a report noting if there are any medical problems and, if so, how they might contribute to the problems found in school. Attention-deficit/hyperactivity disorder is considered to be a medical disability. School professionals might suggest such a diagnosis; however, the diagnosis must be made by a physician. The child's pediatrician must submit a formal report to the school confirming this diagnosis.

When indicated, a mental health evaluation also might be necessary to clarify if there are any psychiatric or emotional problems. If these problems exist, it is necessary to determine whether they are *causing* the academic difficulties or whether they are the secondary *consequence* of the frustrations and failures experienced because of academic difficulties. These assessments will hopefully uncover any contributing family problems as well.

## Conclusion

If the office assessment suggests that a child might have a learning disability, it is important that further studies be done to clarify if this clinical impression is confirmed or if there is another reason for the problems noted.

The timelines from initiation of request until final decisions are made are
- Letter from parent to principal: 10 calendar days
- Initial assessment meeting: 60 calendar days
- Finalizing assessment meeting: done at the final assessment meeting
- IEP finalized (only with parental consent)

## *Bibliography*

US Department of Education. *Building the Legacy: IDEA 2004.* US Department of Education Web site. http://idea.ed.gov/explore/home

Wright PWD, Wright PD. *Wrightslaw: Special Education Law.* Hartfield, VA: Harbor House Law Press; 2008

# PART IV

# Clinical Interventions: The Related Psychiatric Disorders

# Chapter 12

# Interventions for Primary Comorbid Disorders

## Emotional Problems

As previously discussed, it is not uncommon for children and adolescents to have emotional problems reflected by anxiety, depression, or difficulty controlling anger. It is important for the pediatrician to clarify if the presenting emotional problems reflect a specific disorder or a secondary response to emotional, social, or family stress. This chapter will briefly discuss interventions for these primary comorbid disorders.

The clinical presentation of the emotional difficulties is the same whether the difficulties are primary or secondary. It is the history of the disorder that differentiates them. Primary emotional problems relate to underlying brain dysfunction, probably present since birth. Thus there is a chronic and pervasive history of difficulties. The child or adolescent will have experienced similar episodes of difficulty in the past and the difficulties occur in many settings (home, school, with peers, in activities). Often there is a genetic theme with other immediate or extended family members experiencing the same problems. Joseph was 16 when first evaluated. His parents described him as quiet, shy, and "afraid of his shadow." He had no friends and avoided sports and other group activities. His "best friend" was his computer game system. Joseph was aware that he became very nervous around people he did not know or when he had to speak in class. He was also afraid of elevators and being in small, closed spaces. At times he experienced panic attacks during which his heart would race, he would feel sweaty, and he felt like he was going to die. His parents reported that Joseph had been that way since early childhood. His mother admitted that she had the same worries. Joseph did poorly in school. He was in the 11th grade and struggling in each of his classes. On questioning, he described difficulties understanding and retaining what he read. He felt he knew the information, but he could not get his thoughts together to put on a page. Follow-up psychoeducational testing documented that he had learning disabilities that had not previously been identified. By the end of the assessment, it was clear that Joseph had a primary anxiety disorder and learning disabilities.

## Treatment for the Cortically Based Disorders

Interventions for the learning, language, and motor disabilities are discussed in the chapters related to these disorders.

## Treatment for the Emotional Regulatory Problems

Research to date suggests that these emotional regulatory problems are related to a deficiency of a specific neurotransmitter, serotonin, probably in the limbic system. The pharmacologic treatment for anxiety, depression, and anger control disorders is to use one of the selective serotonin reuptake inhibitors (SSRIs) (Table 12-1). Patients respond best when cognitive behavioral therapy is used along with the medication. The focus of this behavioral therapy is to help the child recognize specific feelings and to learn how to control these feelings before they escalate.

For the remainder of this chapter, the medications most frequently used to treat a specific disorder will be noted. It is not the purpose of this book to discuss the dosage and management details when using these medications.

| Table 12-1. Selective Serotonin Reuptake Inhibitors ||
| Trade Name | Generic Name |
| --- | --- |
| Prozac | Fluoxetine |
| Paxil | Paroxetine |
| Zoloft | Sertraline |
| Luvox | Fluvoxamine |
| Celexa | Citalopram |

## FDA "Black Box" Warning for SSRI Use in Children

In 2007 the US Food and Drug Administration issued a black box warning for the use of selective serotonin reuptake inhibitors in children, adolescents, and young adults. The statement included the following:

> Antidepressants increase the risk compared to placebo of suicidal thinking and behavior (suicidality) in children, adolescents, and young adults in short-term studies of major depressive disorder (MDD) and other psychiatric disorders. Anyone considering the use of any antidepressant in a child, adolescent, or young adult must balance this risk with the clinical need. Short-term studies did not show an increase in the risk of suicidality with antidepressants compared to placebo in adults beyond age 24; there was a reduction in risk with antidepressants compared to placebo in adults aged 65 and older. Depression and certain other psychiatric disorders are themselves associated with increases in the risk of suicide. Patients of all ages who are started on antidepressant therapy should be monitored appropriately and observed closely for clinical worsening, suicidality, or unusual changes in behavior. Families and caregivers should be advised of the need for close observation and communication with the prescriber.

## Clinical Alert

Stimulant medications used to treat attention-deficit/hyperactivity disorder (ADHD) may exacerbate an underlying emotional regulatory problem. Whichever problem exists, it becomes clinically worse. We do not know why. For some children, the diagnosis of an anxiety disorder, depression, intermittent explosive disorder, or obsessive-compulsive disorder has been established. However, sometimes, there seems to be a subclinical level of these regulatory problems. The child does not show clinical behaviors reflective of one or more of these disorders. Yet when this child is placed on a stimulant medication, he or she suddenly shows an elevated level of anxiety, depression, anger control difficulty, or obsessive-compulsive behaviors. If the stimulant medication is stopped, these emotional problems decrease or go away. There is a clear relationship between the stimulant medication and the exacerbation of the emotional disorder.

We do not yet understand the interrelationship between the neurochemical difficulties found with ADHD (dopa-dopamine-norepinephrine systems) and the serotonin systems. We do see the clinical picture. Current thinking is that the stimulant medication does not cause these emotional regulatory problems. It is thought that this child has a predisposition for such disorders; however, any symptoms are subclinical. The stimulant medication exacerbates this condition and the symptoms appear. When the stimulant medication is stopped, the behaviors return to a subclinical level.

When this occurs, it is best to treat the regulatory problem with a selective serotonin reuptake inhibitor first. Once under control, the stimulant medication might be reintroduced without difficulty.

## Tic Disorders

Tic disorders are treated if the behaviors are socially embarrassing or if the frequent muscle contractions cause physical discomfort (Table 12-2).

| Table 12-2. Common Medications for Tic Disorders ||
|---|---|
| **Trade Name** | **Generic Name** |
| Catapres | Clonidine |
| Haldol | Haloperidol |
| Tenex | Guanfacine |
| Orap | Pimozide |

New to the treatment of tic disorders is to use one of a group of medications referred to as *atypical antipsychotics.* These are listed in Table 12-3.

| Table 12-3. Atypical Antipsychotics ||
|---|---|
| **Trade Name** | **Generic Name** |
| Risperdal | Risperidone |
| Geodon | Ziprasidone |
| Zyprexa | Olanzapine |
| Seroquel | Quetiapine |
| Abilify | Aripiprazole |

### Clinical Comment

It is known that the use of stimulant medication to treat attention-deficit/hyperactivity disorder might result in the development of tics. The current thinking is not that the stimulant medication "causes" the tics, but that the individual was predisposed to have a tic disorder and the stimulant medication brought it out or exacerbated it. If it is clinically necessary to continue with the stimulant medication, the dose might be lowered and one of the medications to treat the tic disorder added.

# Bipolar Disorders

As discussed in Chapter 8, finalizing the diagnosis of bipolar disorder and establishing a treatment plan is complex. It is best to refer the patient to a child and adolescent psychiatrist to finalize the diagnosis and implement a treatment plan. The pediatrician will continue to see the patient. Thus it is important to keep in contact with this child and adolescent psychiatrist and to know what medications are being used.

The approach to treatment planning will be discussed along with the medications used. This information is to facilitate communication with the child and adolescent psychiatrist. It is not recommended that a pediatrician consider initiating treatment for bipolar disorder.

## Treatment if Depression Is Part of the Clinical Picture

When treating depression, it is important to know that SSRIs frequently exacerbate a bipolar disorder. Sometimes the first clue that the child might have a bipolar disorder is when the clinician notes the chronic and pervasive history of depression and anger control and concludes that the child has an emotional regulatory problem. An SSRI is started and the level of anger and depression increases significantly. Once the SSRI is stopped, these behaviors return to the original level. These reactions suggest that the primary clinical disorder might be a mood disorder, such as bipolar disorder.

To avoid using an SSRI, bupropion (Wellbutrin) will often be used first. The dose needed will vary with the patient. If this medication is not successful, another non-SSRI antidepressant can be tried.

## Treatment if Anger and/or Hypomanic/Manic Behaviors Are Part of the Clinical Picture

No specific medication works for all patients. There are 3 groups of medications that can be used: anticonvulsants, atypical antipsychotics, and lithium. A formal protocol established by the American Academy of Child and Adolescent Psychiatry is followed. First, a medication in one group is tried. If this intervention is not successful, several medications within this group might be tried. If not successful, a medication from another group is considered. Again, if not successful, several medications within this group might be tried. If still not successful, a combination of medications from 2 different groups may be needed.

| Table 12-4. Drugs Commonly Used to Treat Bipolar Disorder ||
|---|---|
| **Anticonvulsant Medications** ||
| **Trade Name** | **Generic** |
| Depakote | Divalproex |
| Tegretol | Carbamazepine |
| Neurontin | Gabapentin |
| Lamictal | Lamotrigine |
| Gabitril | Tiagabine |
| **Atypical Antipsychotic Medications** ||
| Risperdal | Risperidone |
| Zyprexa | Olanzapine |
| Geodon | Ziprasidone |
| Seroquel | Quetiapine |
| Abilify | Aripiprazole |
| **Available Preparations of Lithium** ||
| Eskalith, Lithonate, Lithotabs | Lithium carbonate |
| Lithobid, Eskalith CR | Lithium carbonate slow release |
| Cibalith-S | Lithium citrate syrup |

The medications in each group are listed in Table 12-4. Details on which to use, how to manage, and how to handle any side effects should be addressed by the primary physician for this disorder, the child and adolescent psychiatrist.

## Conclusion

It is essential to be aware of the primary psychiatric disorders that are comorbid with learning disabilities. When a child is diagnosed with a learning disability, it is essential that the pediatrician explore for clinical evidence of any of these other possible comorbid conditions. Unless all existing disorders are recognized, diagnosed, and treated, the child will show a less than complete clinical success.

The pediatrician is in the best situation to recognize the possibility of one or more of these comorbid conditions. Medication management of these comorbid conditions can be challenging. The family, patient, and treating physician need to understand that treating one problem may possibly unmask another underlying condition. In addition, medications are not without side effects.

A pediatrician should consider working with or referring to a child and adolescent psychiatrist for assistance with some of the more difficult situations.

## Bibliography

Silver LB. *The Misunderstood Child. Understanding and Coping with Your Child's Learning Disabilities.* 4th ed. New York, NY: Three Rivers Press; 2006

US Food and Drug Administration. *Antidepressants in Children, Adolescents, and Adults.* US Food and Drug Administration Web site. http://www.fda.gov/Drugs/DrugSafety/InformationbyDrugClass/ucm096273.htm

Chapter 13

# Interventions for the Secondary Emotional, Social, and Family Problems

Monica did not do well in first or second grade. When evaluated, she was 8 years old and 3 months into her third-grade year. Her teacher complained that she never sat still, that she doodled on her papers, and that she had difficulty staying focused on her class work. Her teacher suggested that she might have attention-deficit/hyperactivity disorder (ADHD). Monica's pediatrician prescribed a stimulant medication, but she showed no improvement. She was then referred to a child and adolescent psychiatrist for a consultation. The history showed that neither of the classroom behaviors described by her teacher were noted by her first- or second-grade teachers. Also, starting in October of the current school year, Monica began to be afraid to sleep by herself. She cried unless her mother stayed with her until she was asleep. If she woke up at night, she went to her parents' bedroom. During the day, she became afraid to be in a part of the house if no one else was there. The screening educational assessment showed that her reading and written language skills were at the early second-grade level. Monica admitted that when she could not read the instructions on a worksheet or when she did not know what to write, she became scared that the teacher would be upset with her. Since she could not do the work, she looked around the room while pretending to write. She appeared to be inattentive. Formal studies later confirmed her learning disabilities. Monica's behaviors did not reflect a chronic or a pervasive history of hyperactivity, inattention, or impulsivity. She did not have ADHD. She had unrecognized learning disabilities that resulted in her being anxious in school. Her anxiety resulted in her restless behavior and daydreaming. She was afraid that her parents would find out that she could not do the work and became worried that they would no longer like her. Her separation anxiety increased at home. Her anxiety was secondary to her academic problems. The behaviors caused by her anxiety were misinterpreted as ADHD.

Treatment for Monica must involve addressing both her secondary anxiety disorder and addressing the primary problem: her learning disabilities. This theme is true when planning treatment interventions for any secondary emotional, social, or family problems.

## Treatment for Secondary Emotional Problems

If the emotional, social, or family problems are secondary to the difficulties and frustrations caused by the learning disabilities, it is important to address the learning disabilities early in the intervention process. Is the child recognized as having this disability succeeding in school? Is he or she receiving the necessary services and/or accommodations? Parents must understand the disabilities and how they affect the child and the family. If not, each theme must be addressed.

The interventions needed for the anxiety, depression, anger control difficulties, or other emotional problems are often the same as if these difficulties were considered a primary disability. The unique theme is for the parents, all other relevant adults, the child, and other family members to understand how to use their knowledge of the child's learning abilities and disabilities to understand and help the child.

## Treatment for Secondary Social Problems

Treatment for secondary social problems involves determining whether they are a result of the underlying learning, language, or motor disabilities or if they are also neurologically based.

Parents want to help all of their children grow up with a positive self-image and confidence. These tasks are difficult enough to do with children who have no difficulties. It requires even greater effort and knowledge to help the child who has learning disabilities. It might be easier to excuse this child from chores and other family responsibilities. Such a double standard may communicate a negative message to this child: "We agree that you are inadequate." Such a double standard may cause anger with the other children in the family. "It's not fair. Why do we have to...and he does not?"

Parents must understand their child's areas of learning abilities and disabilities as well as the special education team working with the child at the school. They must understand the disabilities but, more importantly, they must understand the child's abilities. Parents must build on the abilities to select chores, activities, sports, camps, and so many other parts of the child's life. The pediatrician is in an excellent position to help parents understand the child's strengths and weaknesses. The pediatrician can also facilitate having the person who did the assessments or the team working with the child at school to educate parents.

In Chapter 7 a cognitive processing model was outlined to illustrate areas of possible disabilities. This model can be used to teach parents by clarifying both the areas of strength and weakness.

For example, a life profile for 12-year-old Ralph might look like this

| Cognitive Task | Weakness | Strengths |
|---|---|---|
| *Input* | | |
| Visual | Poor visual, fine motor, and visual spatial skills | Good visual motor skills |
| Auditory integration | None | Excellent listening and processing skills |
| Sequencing | Poor motor sequencing skills | Excellent auditory sequencing skills |
| Abstraction | Does not always understand concepts, tasks | Better when verbally explained |
| Organization | Poor with organizing materials, environment, tasks thoughts | Better able to organize |
| *Memory* | | |
| Short-term | Does not always remember tasks, assignments, instructions | Better verbal visual |
| Long-term | None | Good |
| *Output* | | |
| Oral | None | Good |
| Motor | Poor fine motor skills | Good gross motor skills |

Let's use household chores to illustrate how to use this understanding to improve home life. Parents should be able to list their child's strengths and then make another list of their child's weaknesses. Next to the list of strengths they should jot down what chores he or she could do successfully. Next to the list of weaknesses list those chores that might be difficult to do. Next to each of these chores that are difficult for the child, list possible ways a parent might accommodate to allow these chores to be done. (If a parent is stuck, suggest that the special education person in the school or the private tutor help.) For example, if their son has visual motor and fine motor disabilities, it might not be best to ask him to load or unload the dishwasher (unless there are plastic dishes). In place of theses tasks, he could be responsible for walking the dog, bringing in the newspaper, and/or taking out the trash. Each of these tasks requires gross motor skills and minimal eye-hand coordination. Siblings might complain, "It's not fair. Why doesn't he have to do the dishes?" Parents can answer, "Fair does not mean that everybody gets equal. Fair means that each person gets what he or she needs. You can do the dishes. It is difficult for your brother to do them, but he is not being excused. Each of you load the dishwasher once a week and unload once a week. He walks the dog twice a day, brings in the newspaper each day, and takes out the trash each day."

If a child has a sequencing problem and has difficulty setting the dinner table, don't excuse this child from the task. Parents need to learn how to be creative in helping. For example, his mother might say, "Look, I know it is hard for you to set the table because you get confused about where to put the fork, knife, spoon, and glass. So I drew a picture of a typical place setting. I will keep it in this drawer in the kitchen. When it is your turn to set the table, feel free to take it out and use it." What a powerful message this parent is communicating to the child, "You have a disability. I wish you did not. I would do anything to get rid of it, but I can't. I will not excuse you from life, but I will help you learn to compensate and to be successful."

Suppose a young child has sequencing problems and has difficulty getting dressed in the morning. A parent walks in and doesn't know if she should laugh, cry, or be quiet. He has his shirt on and is holding his undershirt. His pants are on but you see the underpants on the floor. Getting the right things on in the right order is not easy. Dressing the child might be fastest but it will not help with self-esteem. Maybe she could lay the clothes for the next day on the floor near the bed or on another bed, putting each item in the order they are to be put on. She puts his favorite teddy bear at the top. Now she can say, "When you get dressed in the morning, start at your teddy bear and work your way down." Maybe this child also has difficulty with the fine motor task of tying shoes. "Bring your shoes downstairs and I will be happy to help you tie them." This child will feel the pride of success because this parent knew how to compensate for his areas of weakness.

The theme is not to excuse the child from any chore or task that is difficult; doing this will continually remind the child that he is inadequate and will create sibling anger. Build on strengths to pick chores they can do. If they must do something that is difficult, try to develop compensatory strategies to facilitate success.

If a child has difficulty with receptive language, parents should be sure to make eye contact with him before speaking. Speak in smaller units and pause at times to ask if he understands. Give one instruction at a time. If it is a set routine, maybe have a written list to give.

How can parents address activities outside of the house to maximize success? What about sports, clubs, and other programs? Again parents must use their knowledge of their child's strengths and weaknesses to select the best activity or to plan the needed adjustments for these activities.

Each sport requires specific skills. Try to pick a sport where the child's strengths match the required skill. For example, if a child has visual perception and visual motor difficulties, she or he might have difficulty with sports that require quick eye-hand coordination—catching, hitting, or throwing a ball. Avoid baseball or basketball if possible. These parents need to look for sports that require more gross motor abilities with minimal eye-hand skills—swimming, soccer, bowling, golf, horseback riding, sailing, canoeing, skiing, certain cross-country and field and track events. If the child resists playing with friends because he cannot play what they are playing, seek a swim team or a bowling league. Let the child make friends there. If playing a sport that is difficult is important to the child, a parent or a private coach might work with the child in private to improve skills. Some children with learning disabilities might have difficulty following directions or understanding strategies, or might play more slowly. They might have trouble remembering the rules of the game or the sequence of a particular drill.

With all sports activities, it is important that the coach understand the child's areas of strength and weakness. Such knowledge leads to picking the right position and understanding how to be understanding and supportive.

The same approach is used with all outside activities. Build on strengths; don't magnify weaknesses. For example, picture a 10-year-old girl with fine motor, sequencing, and visual motor disabilities at a Girl Scout meeting. Everyone is working on a project, maybe drawing and cutting out a turkey for the Thanksgiving celebration. This child's cutouts or drawings are not very good. She cannot color and stay within the lines or cut and stay on the line. Everybody laughs and teases. Another failure, and this child does not want to go to any more meetings. But if the parents met with the activity leader early in the year and explained their daughter's strengths and weaknesses, the scout leader could have handled it differently. At the meeting prior to this one, the leader might have said to this girl, "Next month we are going to cut out turkeys. Would you read about why the turkey is the symbol for Thanksgiving and be prepared to explain it to the group?" Now the meeting comes around. Everyone else is doing their fine motor tasks. This girl is standing up and verbally explaining why the turkey is the symbol. She is successful and the evening is saved.

Parents must think in this way for every aspect of their child's life. Pick the activities that build on strengths. Educate all who need to know about the weaknesses and how to avoid or compensate for them. Sunday school teachers, piano teachers, martial arts instructors—all need to understand if they are to help.

Selection of day and summer camps is no exception. Does this child need a noncompetitive, non-sports camp? What activities might be difficult? Parents need to speak with the camp directors and specific counselors to be sure they understand how to build on strengths and not magnify weaknesses.

What about siblings? If the child with learning disabilities is excused from responsibilities or if a parent must do more for this child, siblings will get angry. "It's not fair!!" If this child acts inappropriately in the neighborhood, on the school bus, or at school, siblings will be embarrassed and get angry. If they do not know about their sibling's learning disability, they might wonder why he or she is in a special class or goes to a different school.

Parents need to learn how to explain to their other children. They need to know how to speak to the strengths as well as the difficulties. They need to explain what is being done to help.

So whether it is home life, sports, activities, or camps, parents play a major role in helping their child succeed within the family, in activities, and socially. To do this, it is critical that these parents learn their child's areas of learning disabilities and learning abilities. Without this knowledge, they will not know how to build on the strengths and to compensate or accommodate for the weaknesses.

Ideally the professional who did the testing or the special education team working with the child will help the parents to learn. If this has not helped, the pediatrician can facilitate connecting the parents with someone who can help them learn.

## Conclusion

Secondary emotional, social, and family problems must be addressed through psychological help, possibly with medication. But these efforts will not be successful unless the primary stressor causing these problems is addressed: the learning disabilities. The pediatrician must assist in confirming the diagnosis and in ensuring that the child receives the necessary help. In addition to these professional services, parents play an important role in addressing disabilities. It is essential that parents understand their child's areas of learning abilities and disabilities. With this knowledge they can learn to use the child's strengths and compensate for or avoid tasks or activities that involve the child's weaknesses. This concept is equally true for other adults who interact with the child—coaches, teachers, group leaders. The pediatrician can and should play an important role in facilitating this educational process and supporting the child and his or her family.

## Bibliography

Silver LB. *The Misunderstood Child. Understanding and Coping with Your Child's Learning Disabilities.* 4th ed. New York, NY: Three Rivers Press; 2006

# PART V

# Resources

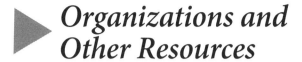

# *Organizations and Other Resources*

## Organizations Related to Learning Disabilities

### *Learning Disabilities Association of America (LDA)*

4156 Library Rd
Pittsburgh, PA 15234
412/341-1515
www.ldaamerica.org

A national volunteer-run, nonprofit organization with state and local chapters. Membership is open to parents, individuals with learning disabilities, educators, and health and mental health professionals. LDA advocates for individuals with learning disabilities and their families, provides direct help to individuals and families, provides literature and other resources, offers national and state conferences, and encourages research on learning disabilities. Through its Healthy Children Project, it works to inform people of the concerns with environmental toxins and the possible impact these toxins have on the child. By contacting the national office on the Web site, it is possible to contact state and local chapters.

### *National Center for Learning Disabilities*

381 Park Ave South, Suite 1401
New York, NY 10016
888/575-7373
www.ncld.org

A national nonprofit organization that offers information, develops and conducts educational programs, raises public awareness of learning disabilities, and advocates for improved legislation and services for those with learning disabilities.

### International Dyslexia Association
Chester Building, Suite 382
8600 LaSalle Rd
Baltimore, MD 21286
800/222-3123
www.interdys.org

An international nonprofit membership organization that offers training in language-based programs and provides publications relating to dyslexia. There are chapters in most states.

### LDonline
Ldonline/WETA TV
2775 South Quincy St
Arlington, VA 22206
703/998-2825
www.LDonline.com

An excellent Web site for parents and professionals providing information and resources relating to learning disabilities.

### National Institute of Child Health and Human Development
NICHD Information Resource Center
PO Box 3006
Rockville, MD 20847
800/370-2943
www.nichd.nih.gov

An institute within the National Institutes of Health that sponsors research in learning disabilities. It provides reviews of literature and information.

### Office of Special Education and Rehabilitative Services
US Department of Education
400 Maryland Ave, SW
Washington, DC 20202
800/872-5327
www.ed.gov.osers

A federal office providing information about special education programs, vocational rehabilitation programs, and national/international research.

# Professional Organizations

### American Academy of Child and Adolescent Psychiatry
3615 Wisconsin Ave, NW
Washington, DC 20016
aacap.org

### American Academy of Ophthalmology
1101 Vermont Ave, NW
Washington, DC 20036
aao.org

### American Academy of Optometry
5530 Wisconsin Ave
Chevy Chase, MD 20815
aaopt.org

### American Academy of Pediatrics
141 Northwest Point Blvd
Elk Grove Village, IL 60007
www.aap.org

### American Medical Association
515 North State St
Chicago, IL 60610
www.ama-assn.org

### American Occupational Therapy Association
PO Box 31220
Bethesda, MD 20824
aota.org

### American Psychiatric Association
1000 Wilson Blvd, Suite 1825
Arlington, VA 22209
psych.org

### American Psychological Association
750 First St, NE
Washington, DC 20002
apa.org

### American Speech, Language, and Hearing Association
2200 Research Blvd
Rockville, MD 20850
asha.org

### National Association of School Psychologists
4340 East West Highway, Suite 402
Bethesda, MD 20814
nasponline.org

### National Association of Social Workers
7981 Eastern Ave
Silver Spring, MD 20910
naswdc.org

# Screening Forms

Patient's Name: _____

Date of Birth: _____ Today's Date: _____

Grade in School: _____

## Learning Disabilities Screening Questions

(Note: This questionnaire is meant merely to screen for the possibility of learning disabilities. Further evaluation would be required for diagnosis.)

**To be completed by the parent/guardian (and/or reworded for older children). Please check the answer that best applies to your child.**

### All Children

Have there been any concerns noted on your child's report card?

☐ No Concerns Noted          ☐ Yes, Academic Concerns
☐ Yes, Behavior Concerns     ☐ Yes, Academic and Behavior Concerns

|  | Never | Sometimes | Often |
|---|---|---|---|
| Are there struggles over completing homework? | ☐ | ☐ | ☐ |

Do you and your child see the homework as being: ☐ Too Hard  ☐ Too Easy  ☐ Just Right

### Preschool/Kindergarten

|  |  | Never | Sometimes | Often |
|---|---|---|---|---|
| **Reading:** | Can your child recognize letters and numbers? | ☐ | ☐ | ☐ |
|  | Does your child know the sounds that each letter makes? | ☐ | ☐ | ☐ |
| **Writing:** | Does your child have difficulties with coloring or cutting? | ☐ | ☐ | ☐ |
|  | Is your child learning to form letters and numbers? | ☐ | ☐ | ☐ |
| **Math:** | Is your child beginning to understand numbers and their meaning? | ☐ | ☐ | ☐ |
|  | Can your child count to 10? | ☐ | ☐ | ☐ |

Please explain any "sometimes" or "often" answers: _____

**Learning Disabilities Screening Questions (page 2)** Patient's Name: _____

Date of Birth: _____/Today's Date: _____

## First/Second Grade

| | | Never | Sometimes | Often |
|---|---|---|---|---|
| **Reading:** | Can your child sound out words? | ☐ | ☐ | ☐ |
| | Does your child recognize words learned earlier in the year? | ☐ | ☐ | ☐ |
| | Is your child reading at the level of the other children? | ☐ | ☐ | ☐ |
| **Writing:** | Can your child form all letters and numbers? | ☐ | ☐ | ☐ |
| | Does your child write on the line? | ☐ | ☐ | ☐ |
| **Math:** | Has your child mastered addition of single digits? | ☐ | ☐ | ☐ |
| | Has your child mastered subtraction of single digits? | ☐ | ☐ | ☐ |

Please explain any "sometimes" or "often" answers:_____

_____

_____

## Third/Fourth Grade

| | | Never | Sometimes | Often |
|---|---|---|---|---|
| **Reading:** | Does your child understand what he or she reads? | ☐ | ☐ | ☐ |
| | Does your child enjoy reading? | ☐ | ☐ | ☐ |
| **Writing:** | Has your child learned to capitalize? | ☐ | ☐ | ☐ |
| | Has your child learned to use punctuation correctly? | ☐ | ☐ | ☐ |
| | Does your child spell as well as the teacher expects him to? | ☐ | ☐ | ☐ |
| | Can your child write full sentence answers on assignments? | ☐ | ☐ | ☐ |
| **Math:** | If it has been covered in class, can your child do multiplication and division problems? | ☐ | ☐ | ☐ |
| | If it has been covered in class, can your child do math with fractions and decimals? | ☐ | ☐ | ☐ |
| | Are your child's math skills at the level expected by the teacher? | ☐ | ☐ | ☐ |

**Learning Disabilities Screening Questions (page 3)**     Patient's Name: _____

Date of Birth: _____/Today's Date: _____

## Third/Fourth Grade (continued)

Please explain any "sometimes" or "often" answers: _____

_____

_____

## Fifth Grade and Middle School

| | | Never | Sometimes | Often |
|---|---|---|---|---|
| **Reading:** | Can your child read with ease and understand what is read? | ☐ | ☐ | ☐ |
| | Does your child retain the information from reading? | ☐ | ☐ | ☐ |
| **Writing:** | Can your child organize thoughts and get them down on the page? | ☐ | ☐ | ☐ |
| | Do your child's teachers think his answers to questions and assignments are complete and fully addressing the material? | ☐ | ☐ | ☐ |
| **Math:** | Are your child's math skills at grade level? | ☐ | ☐ | ☐ |
| | Can your child do calculations without making too many careless errors? | ☐ | ☐ | ☐ |
| **Organization:** | Are your child's papers, notebooks, and backpack neat and organized? | ☐ | ☐ | ☐ |
| | Is your child's desk, locker, bedroom organized? | ☐ | ☐ | ☐ |
| | Does your child lose, forget, or misplace papers and other materials? | ☐ | ☐ | ☐ |
| | Does your child have difficulty organizing information when studying for tests or writing papers? | ☐ | ☐ | ☐ |
| **Executive Function:** | Is your child good at planning out how to do homework assignments? | ☐ | ☐ | ☐ |
| | Does your child get work done on time? | ☐ | ☐ | ☐ |

Please explain any "sometimes" or "often" answers: _____

_____

_____

**Learning Disabilities Screening Questions (page 4)**    Patient's Name: _____

Date of Birth: _____/Today's Date: _____

## High School

| | | Never | Sometimes | Often |
|---|---|:---:|:---:|:---:|
| **Reading:** | Can your teen keep up with the reading demands of each class? | ☐ | ☐ | ☐ |
| | Can your teen use the material he reads to answer questions? | ☐ | ☐ | ☐ |
| | Do you notice that your teen might misread questions or instructions on assignments? | ☐ | ☐ | ☐ |
| **Writing:** | Does your teen have difficulty writing the correct response to questions? | ☐ | ☐ | ☐ |
| | Can your teen write a report that covers everything the teacher wanted? | ☐ | ☐ | ☐ |
| | Do you find that you have to help your teen organize his/her thoughts before he/she can write a paper? | ☐ | ☐ | ☐ |
| **Math:** | Does your teen sometimes misread a word problem? | ☐ | ☐ | ☐ |
| | Is your teen succeeding in learning the math concepts that are being taught? | ☐ | ☐ | ☐ |
| | Does your teen make careless errors when doing calculations? | ☐ | ☐ | ☐ |
| **Organization:** | Are your teen's papers, notebooks, and backpack neat and organized? | ☐ | ☐ | ☐ |
| | Is your teen's desk, locker, bedroom organized? | ☐ | ☐ | ☐ |
| | Does your teen lose, forget, or misplace papers and other materials? | ☐ | ☐ | ☐ |
| | Does your teen have difficulty organizing information when studying for tests or writing papers? | ☐ | ☐ | ☐ |
| **Executive Function:** | Is your teen good at planning out how to do homework assignments? | ☐ | ☐ | ☐ |
| | Does your teen get work done on time? | ☐ | ☐ | ☐ |

Please explain any "sometimes" or "often" answers:_____

_____

Patient's Name: _____

Date of Birth: _____  Today's Date: _____

# Language Disabilities Screening Questions

(Note: This questionnaire is meant merely to screen for the possibility of language disabilities. Further evaluation would be required for diagnosis.)

**To be completed by the parent/guardian (and/or reworded for older children). Please check the answer that best applies to your child.**

### *Receptive Language*

| | Never | Sometimes | Often |
|---|---|---|---|
| Do you find that it helps to have eye contact when you speak to your child? | ☐ | ☐ | ☐ |
| Do you notice that you need to speak slower or need to focus on getting your child's attention before you can ask him/her a question? | ☐ | ☐ | ☐ |
| Can you give more than one instruction at a time? | ☐ | ☐ | ☐ |
| Do teachers say that your child has trouble following spoken instructions in class? | ☐ | ☐ | ☐ |
| Does your child understand figures of speech (such as irony or metaphors)? | ☐ | ☐ | ☐ |
| Does your child understand jokes and/or sarcasm? | ☐ | ☐ | ☐ |

### *Expressive Language*

| | Never | Sometimes | Often |
|---|---|---|---|
| When your child initiates a conversation, does he have any problems finding the right words to express himself? | ☐ | ☐ | ☐ |
| When you ask your child a question, does he sometimes struggle to find the right words or have trouble organizing his thoughts when he responds? | ☐ | ☐ | ☐ |
| Is it hard to get a conversation going with your child? | ☐ | ☐ | ☐ |

## Questions to ask of an older child

### *Receptive Language*

| | Never | Sometimes | Often |
|---|---|---|---|
| When the teacher is speaking in class, do you sometimes have trouble understanding or keeping up with what is being said? | ☐ | ☐ | ☐ |
| Do you sometimes find that you misunderstand what people are saying and give the wrong answer or response? | ☐ | ☐ | ☐ |

**Language Disabilities Screening Questions (page 2)**     Patient's Name: _____

Date of Birth: _____/Today's Date: _____

When people are talking, do you find that you have to focus
    so hard on what they are saying that you sometimes fall
    behind and miss what is being said?    ☐    ☐    ☐

If the teacher talks too much, do you get lost and not fully
    understand what is being said?    ☐    ☐    ☐

## *Expressive Language*

Do you find that sometimes you have trouble getting
    your thoughts together when you have to answer
    a question?    ☐    ☐    ☐

Do you find that sometimes you can't find the words you
    want to use when you are talking at home, at school, or
    with your friends?    ☐    ☐    ☐

Please explain any "sometimes" or "often" answers: _____

_____

_____

Patient's Name: _____

Date of Birth: _____ Today's Date: _____

# Motor Coordination Screening Questions

(Note: This questionnaire is meant merely to screen for the possibility of motor disabilities. Further evaluation would be required for diagnosis.)

**To be completed by the parent/guardian (and/or reworded for older children). Please check the answer that best applies to your child.**

## Fine motor/gross motor questions

*Preschool/Kindergarten*

| | Never | Sometimes | Often |
|---|---|---|---|
| 1. Does your child have difficulty with coloring or cutting? | ☐ | ☐ | ☐ |
| 2. Does your child have difficulty with buttoning, zipping, or tying? | ☐ | ☐ | ☐ |
| 3. Can your child manage the fork, knife, and spoon when eating? | ☐ | ☐ | ☐ |
| 4. Does your child prefer to eat with his fingers? | ☐ | ☐ | ☐ |
| 5. Can your child run, jump, skip, climb as well as his or her friends? | ☐ | ☐ | ☐ |
| 6. Does your child knock things over or bump into things a lot? | ☐ | ☐ | ☐ |

*Elementary School and Older*

| | Never | Sometimes | Often |
|---|---|---|---|
| 1. Is your child's handwriting neat enough? | ☐ | ☐ | ☐ |
| 2. Is your child's handwriting fast enough? | ☐ | ☐ | ☐ |
| 3. When playing sports, is your child coordinated? | ☐ | ☐ | ☐ |
| 4. Does your child have difficulty with catching, hitting, throwing? | ☐ | ☐ | ☐ |
| 5. When you watch your child run, does he seem to be as coordinated and as fast as other children his age? | ☐ | ☐ | ☐ |

Please explain any "sometimes" or "often" answers: _____

_____

**Motor Coordination Screening Questions (page 2)**     Patient's Name: _____

Date of Birth: _____ /Today's Date: _____

## Tactile Questions

|  | Never | Sometimes | Often |
|---|---|---|---|
| 1. Is your child sensitive to clothing? | ☐ | ☐ | ☐ |
| 2. Does your child complain about tags, elastic, socks, or the texture of clothes? | ☐ | ☐ | ☐ |
| 3. Does your child like to be held and cuddled? | ☐ | ☐ | ☐ |
| 4. Did your child like to be held and cuddled as an infant? | ☐ | ☐ | ☐ |
| 5. Is your child more sensitive to loud noises than others? | ☐ | ☐ | ☐ |
| 6. Is your child more sensitive to smells, tastes, and textures of foods than others? | ☐ | ☐ | ☐ |

Please explain any "sometimes" or "often" answers: _____

_____

_____

_____

_____

_____

## Vestibular Questions

|  | Never | Sometimes | Often |
|---|---|---|---|
| 1. Can your child ride (older than age 5 or 6) a two-wheel bike? | ☐ | ☐ | ☐ |
| 2. Can your child go up and down steps in tandem (alternating his or her feet)? | ☐ | ☐ | ☐ |
| 3. Does your child like to rest his or her head on an arm, or to lean, slump down, or lie down when sitting at a desk? | ☐ | ☐ | ☐ |

Please explain any "sometimes" or "often" answers: _____

_____

_____

_____

_____

_____

# *Index*